APHA MISSION STATEMENT

The American Public Health Association is an association of individuals and organizations working to improve the public's health. It promotes the scientific and professional foundation of public health practice and policy, advocates the conditions for a healthy global society, emphasizes prevention, and enhances the ability of members to promote and protect environmental and community health.

American Public Health Association
800 I St., NW
Washington, DC 20001-3710

Mohammad N. Akhter, MD, MPH
Executive Director

APHA Publications Board Liasons: Don Jaco, Basil Vareldzis

Printed and bound in the United States of America
Set In: Garamond
Printed and bound in the United States of America
Interior Design and Typesetting: Joseph R. Loehle
Cover Design: Joseph R. Loehle
Printing and Binding: United Book Press

ISBN 0-87553-027-3
2 M 9/02

Communicating
PUBLIC HEALTH
INFORMATION
Effectively

A Guide For Practitioners

David E. Nelson, MD, MPH
Ross C. Brownson, PhD
Patrick L. Remington, MD, MPH
Claudia Parvanta, PhD
Editors

table of contents

ACKNOWLEDGEMENTS   ix

CONTRIBUTORS   xi

FOREWORD   xv

PREFACE   xvii

PART I: BACKGROUND AND FRAMEWORK

CHAPTER 1: CURRENT ISSUES AND CHALLENGES   1

Background
Barriers to Communication
The Field of Health Communication
Summary

CHAPTER 2: PUBLIC HEALTH COMMUNICATION: 11
A PLANNING FRAMEWORK

Background
Public Health Communication Framework
Examples of Applying the Public Health Communication Planning Framework
Summary

CHAPTER 3: TRANSLATING PUBLIC HEALTH DATA   33

Background
Locating Public Health Data and Other Scientific Information
Translating Public Health Data: General Considerations
Translating Public Health Data: Recommended Formats
Challenges and Barriers
Summary

PART II: AUDIENCES

CHAPTER 4: GENERAL PUBLIC: COMMUNICATING TO INFORM   47

Background
Getting to Know the Audience
Information Processing
Message Development and Planning
Challenges and Barriers
Summary

CHAPTER 5: GENERAL PUBLIC: COMMUNICATING TO PERSUADE 59
Background
Overview of Persuasive Health Communication Approaches and Theories
Purpose and Audience
Message Development, Media and Channel Selection, and Evaluation
Summary

CHAPTER 6: COMMUNICATING PUBLIC HEALTH INFORMATION 73
TO THE NEWS MEDIA
Background
Purpose, Audience, and Message
Message Production, Delivery, and Timing
General Characteristics and Recommendations for Communicating with the News Media
Specific Recommendations for Communicating with the News Media
Media Advocacy
Challenges and Barriers
Summary

CHAPTER 7: COMMUNICATING PUBLIC HEALTH INFORMATION 97
TO POLICY MAKERS
Background
Characteristics of Policy Makers
Purpose, Audience, and Message
Selecting a Spokesperson and Message Production and Delivery
General Recommendations for Communicating with Policy Makers
Additional Recommendations for Communicating with Elected Officials
Challenges and Barriers
Summary

CHAPTER 8: COMMUNICATING PUBLIC HEALTH INFORMATION 115
TO PRIVATE AND VOLUNTARY HEALTH ORGANIZATIONS
Background
Types of Private and Voluntary Health Organizations
Rationale for Communicating Information to Private and Voluntary Health Organizations
Purpose, Audience, and Message
Suggested Types of Public Health Data to Communicate
Negotiating an Exchange
Challenges and Barriers
Summary

PART III: MESSAGE DELIVERY
CHAPTER 9: WRITTEN COMMUNICATION 127
Background
Types of Written Materials Used in Public Health Communication
Purpose, Audience, and Message
General Recommendations for Written Communication
Specific Recommendations for Written Communication
Writing for Low Literacy Audiences
Summary

CHAPTER 10: ORAL PRESENTATIONS 141
Background
Characteristics of Oral Presentations
Additional Recommendations for Improving Oral Presentations
Challenges and Barriers
Summary

CHAPTER 11: VISUAL COMMUNICATION   **155**

Background
General Considerations
Purpose, Audience, and Message
Specific Visual Communication Modalities
Other Considerations for Visual Communication
Challenges and Barriers
Summary

CHAPTER 12: ELECTRONIC COMMUNICATION   **173**

Background
General Considerations for Electronic Communication in Public Health
Purpose, Audience, and Message
Specific Recommendations for E-mail
Specific Recommendations for Web Sites
Limitations of Electronic Communication
Summary

CHAPTER 13: RISK COMMUNICATION   **185**

Background
Risk Perception
Purpose, Audience, and Message
Message Production and Delivery
Recommendations for Risk Communication
Challenges and Barriers
Risk Communication Planning
Bioterrorism and Communication
Summary

PART IV: NEXT STEPS

CHAPTER 14: FUTURE DIRECTIONS   **205**

Introduction
Increased Health Communication Education and Training
Increased Health Communication Research
Improved Translation of Existing Public Health Information
Enhanced Tailoring of Messages and Increased Use of Multiple Mass Media Channels
Improved Cultural Communication Competency
Building Infrastructure for Equitable Access and Use of New Communication Technologies
Conclusion

APPENDIX 1: STEP-BY-STEP PLANNING GUIDE FOR   **213**
COMMUNICATING PUBLIC HEALTH INFORMATION

APPENDIX 2: DIRECTORIES AND OTHER SELECTED INTERNET   **215**
WEB SITES FOR LOCATING PUBLIC HEALTH DATA

APPENDIX 3: INTERNET WEB SITES FOR STATES AND THE   **221**
DISTRICT OF COLUMBIA

INDEX   **225**

acknowledgements

This book would not have been possible without the assistance of many people. In particular, we thank Natoshia Askelson, Don Austin, B. Sue Bell, R. Elliott Churchill, Karen Davis, Barbara Dougherty, Ellen Eisner, David Espey, David Fleming, Shelley Foster, Vickie Freimuth, Tammie Gilbert, Jeannie Herrera, Gary Hogelin, Jim Holt, Phil Huang, Rick Hull, Denise Jackson, Susan Kirby, Gary Kreps, Marshall Kreuter, Barbara Levine, Dan Longo, Anne Lubenow, Marcia Mabee, James S. Marks, Chris Maylahn, Brenda Mazzocchi, Jim Mendlein, Viviane McKay, Ali Mokdad, Claire Nelson, Hayley Nelson, Patrick O'Carroll, Linda Williams Pickle, Chris Prue, Gloria Rasband, Mike Rothschild, Nancy Silver, Eduardo Simoes, Carol Stanwyck, Emma Stupp, Sue Stableford, Peter Taylor, Katie Trout, and the anonymous APHA reviewers for their contributions. We especially thank Stephanie Renna for her help with graphics.

DEN
RCB
PLR
CP

contributors

David Ahrens, MA
Research Program Manager
Tobacco Monitoring and Evalution Program
University of Wisconsin Comprehensive Cancer Center
Madison, WI

Elaine Bratic Arkin, BA
Health Communications Consultant
Arlington, VA

Ross C. Brownson, PhD
Professor of Epidemiology and Chair
Department of Community Health
Saint Louis University School of Public Health
Salus Center
St. Louis, MO

Tom Eng, VMD, MPH
President
eHealth Institute
Silver Spring, MD

Carmelle Goldberg, MSc
Researcher
Régie Régionale de la Santé et des Services Sociaux
Direction de la Santé Publique de Montréal-Centre
Montreal, Canada

Michael Greenwell, BA
Associate Director for Communications
National Center for Chronic Disease Prevention and Health Promotion
Centers for Disease Prevention and Control (CDC)
Atlanta, GA

Isaac Lipkus, PhD
Associate Research Professor
Duke University Medical Center
Durham, NC

Max Lum, EdD, MPA
Associate Director for Health Communications
National Institute for Occupational Safety and Health
Centers for Disease Control and Prevention
Washington, DC

Edward Maibach, MPH, PhD
Worldwide Director of Social Marketing
Porter Novelli
Washington, DC

Bernard R. Malone, MPA
Director, Division of Chronic Disease Prevention & Health Promotion
Missouri Department of Health and Senior Services
Jefferson City, MO

Dianne L. Needham, MPA, PE
Deputy Director, Communications
Warren Grant Magnuson Clinical Center
National Institutes of Health
Bethesda, MD

David E. Nelson, MD, M.H
Senior Health Scientist
Health Communication and Informatics Research Branch
Behavioral Research Program
Division of Cancer Control and Population Sciences
National Cancer Institute
Bethesda, MD

Claudia Parvanta, PhD
Director, Division of Health Communication
Office of Communication
Centers for Disease Prevention and Control
Atlanta, GA

J. Gregory Payne, PhD
Director
Center for Ethics in Political and Health Communication
Emerson College
Boston, MA

Scott C. Ratzan, MD, MPA, MA
Vice President, Government Relaions, Europe
Johnson & Johnson
St. Stevens-Woluwe, Belgium
Editor, Journal of Health Communication
Academy for the Advancement of Health, LLC.
Washington, DC

Patrick L. Remington, MD, MPH
Associate Professor
Department of Population Health Sciences
Director, Public Health and Health Policy Institute
University of Wisconsin School of Medicine
Madison, WI

Lee Ann Riesenberg, RN, MS
Director, Medical Education
Guthrie/Robert Packer Hospital
Sayre, PA

Paul Z. Siegel, MD, MPH
Director, Field Epidemilogy Program
National Center for Chronic Disease Prevention and Health Promotion
Centers for Disease Prevention and Control (CDC)
Atlanta, GA

Tim L. Tinker, DrPH, MPH
Vice President, Science and Health
Widmeyer Communications
Washington DC

Elaine Vaughan, PhD
Associate Professor
Department of Psychology and Social Behavior, School of Social Ecology
University of California, Irvine
Irvine, CA

Jennifer A. Woodward, PhD
State Registrar/Manager
Center for Health Statistics
Oregon Department of Human Services
Portland, OR

foreword

In this age of information, the need for public health practitioners to communicate information to nonscientific audiences such as the general public, the news media, and policy makers has never been greater. The importance of health communication was never more evident than during the anthrax attacks of October 2001. Translating health information effectively at both the individual and societal level is essential for reducing mortality and morbidity, as well as for improving the quality of life.

The past century saw dramatic shifts in many areas of public health, with the most obvious being the shift in the causes of death and disability. In 1900, the major causes of death were infectious diseases such as pneumonia, tuberculosis, and diarrhea. In the 21st century, we face heart disease, cancer, stroke, and injury. The implications of these shifts for public health practice are equally dramatic.

Of course, the prevention and control of infectious diseases such as pneumonia and tuberculosis have always involved the need to communicate information to those at risk. For chronic diseases and injury, many of which are preventable through individual behavior change or through policy, environmental, or clinical interventions, communication is equally, if not more, important. Simple precautions such as cooking meat to an adequate temperature can eliminate the risk of certain deadly food-borne illnesses, yet those of us in public health are well aware that there is a large difference between what is known by scientists and what is actually practiced among the general population. For example, although the recommendation for routine breast cancer screening began in the 1970s, it took nearly 20 years before half of all women were compliant. These differences clearly speak to the need for improved communication with the public and with policy makers.

As the first of its kind, this book provides a comprehensive approach to help public health practitioners in both the public and private sectors to improve their ability to communicate with different audiences. From the news media to legislators, and from visual communication to electronic communication, every chapter provides practical, real-world recommendations and examples of how to communicate public health information to nonscientific audiences more effectively. The knowledge and skills gleaned from this book will assist with planning and executing the communication activities commonly done by public health professionals.

The communications environment at the dawn of the 21st century has been frequently described as cluttered. Thousands of messages are sent every day encouraging people to buy this, do that, and act now. In order to compete in this increasingly competitive and complex environment, those of us in public health must make the science and art of communication as integral a part of our everyday activities as the science of epidemiology and disease control. I believe this book provides an important first step towards that end.

Jeffrey P. Koplan, M.D., M.P.H.
Vice President for Academic Health Affairs
Emory University

preface

The need for this book became clear to the authors based on their own daily work in public health practice and in discussions with professional colleagues. Most of the epidemiology literature, for example, focuses on research methods or the determinants of specific diseases or health risk factors, not on how to disseminate or use epidemiologic information in public health practice.

In schools of public health and other health professional institutions, practitioners receive little formal training on communicating with persons outside the scientific community. These nonscientific audiences include the general public, the news media, policy makers, voluntary health organizations, and private health organizations. The skills needed to communicate with such audiences are usually learned (if learned at all) only after years of experience. In marked contrast, the discipline of health communication strongly emphasizes the need to understand nonscientific audiences and to develop materials tailored to their needs. Whether trying to encouraging individual behavior change or advocating for policy, we strongly believe that public health professionals can greatly benefit from applying knowledge from the field of health communication to their communication efforts.

The growing interest in health and the ongoing improvement in information technology provide unprecedented communication opportunities for public health practitioners. The purpose of this book is to provide practical information to help practitioners better understand nonscientific audiences and how to communicate information to them through various means. The book is intended for communication that occurs in many situations, ranging from a one-on-one meeting with a high-level administrator, to working through the news media or the Internet to reach mass audiences.

The book attempts to strike a balance between science and practical recommendations. For some areas, such as communicating with the general public, there is a substantial body of scientific research; for others, such as communicating with policy makers or using electronic communication, the research is limited. The book is designed to be used primarily as a primer to help those who need background information or guidance when faced with specific communication situations.

This book is intended for several audiences. It can be used by practicing local, state, or national public health professionals in the private or public sector, including epidemiologists, health educators, health promotion specialists, environmental/occupational health specialists, administrators, physicians, nurses, dentists, veterinarians, and sanitarians to improve their communication with nonscientific audiences. Professionals involved in the teaching of public health will find the book of value for introducing the practical side of translating public health information into public health action. The book will be valuable for public health students to help broaden their vision of the practice of public health.

The authors of the chapters were selected based both on their scientific expertise and their experience in public health practice or health communication. All authors have many years of practical experience in communicating public health information to nonscientific audiences.

The topics in this book underscore the multidisciplinary nature of public health communication. The first chapter describes reasons why practitioners often fail to communicate with nonscientific audiences and how knowledge based on the field of health communication can and improve this situation. Chapter 2 provides the framework for communicating public health information used throughout the book. It introduces the need to consider the purpose (why), audience (who), message (what), media and channels for message delivery (how/where), timing (when), and evaluation. Chapter 3 covers translating data for nonscientific audiences.

Chapters 4 through 8 are the audience chapters, and they review the characteristics and communication considerations for addressing the general public, news media, policy makers, voluntary health organizations, and private health organizations. Chapters 9 through 12 describe different aspects of message delivery, and include written, oral, visual, and electronic communication. Chapter 13 covers the challenging area of risk communication. Although presented as separate chapters, the material in chapter 4 through 8 and chapters 9 through 13 are strongly interrelated. Finally, the last chapter suggests future directions for improving public health communication.

A standard format has been used for most chapters to improve consistency, and to allow readers quick and rapid access to desired information. This format consists of a brief introduction to the chapter, background information, and recommended approaches. A short list of suggested readings and resources is also supplied for readers to help locate additional relevant material. Practical examples are used to illustrate important key points. Although designed to be read in its entirety, except for chapters 4 and 5 each chapter can be read independently, thus facilitating use by readers who need specific information when preparation time is limited.

This book is not designed to be the definitive work on public health communication, as this field is broad. The topics addressed in each chapter could easily be developed into entire books, indeed, many already have been. Much has been written, for example, on written communication, oral presentations, risk communication, and informing or persuading general public audiences. Instead, we have tried to summarize what we consider to be the essential information for the most common communication situations and challenges faced by practitioners.

The need for collaboration between health communicators and public health practitioners has never been greater, and it is our goal to help make this a reality. We hope this book will be a useful resource for practitioners as they strive to improve the health of individuals and of our society through improved communication of public health information.

August 2002

David E. Nelson, MD, MPH
Ross C. Brownson, PhD
Patrick L. Remington, MD, MPH
Claudia Parvanta, PhD

Part I:

Background and Framework

Chapter One

CURRENT ISSUES AND CHALLENGES

David E. Nelson, MD, MPH

Public health practitioners spend a substantial amount of time and effort learning the skills necessary to perform their jobs. These skills are commonly learned through formal coursework in universities, continuing education, on-the-job training, mentoring, or experience. Scientists and other public health professionals may spend years learning the methods to collect, analyze, and interpret data, but most receive little training on communicating information. For effective public health practice, information must be appropriately communicated to diverse audiences, most of which consist of individuals outside the scientific community.[1,2]

Consider the importance of communicating public health information in each of the following scenarios:

- At 4:30 pm on a Friday, a call is received from a newspaper reporter about a suspected food-borne illness among persons who have eaten hamburger at a well-known restaurant chain.[3] The reporter wants to know how many people have been affected and what the risk is for others who have eaten hamburger at the chain's restaurants.

- The state public health association is actively supporting efforts to reduce smoking by increasing state excise taxes on tobacco. Expecting a tough struggle against the tobacco lobby, the association seeks the support of a major health organization, but the organization first asks for strong evidence that the tax increase will decrease smoking.[4]

- A published report suggests an increased risk of breast cancer in the local community, and many residents are convinced that chemicals from a nearby factory are the cause.[5] A public hearing is scheduled at which public health professionals will discuss the risk to the community.

• A new governor has pledged to reduce state spending by cutting resources for programs that promote immoral behaviors. In his efforts to address a state budget deficit, the governor has proposed a drastic reduction in program funds for sexually transmitted disease (STD) prevention. The director of the state health department decides to present information on the effectiveness of the STD program to a high-level administrator, who is a recent political appointee of the governor with no health experience.

These scenarios demonstrate the importance that communication outside the health community plays in furthering public health goals. Translating public health information is essential to increase knowledge, facilitate informed decision-making, or encourage change among individuals and policy makers. With the explosion of interest in public health topics over the past several decades, the days when practitioners could focus solely on interacting with health professionals are gone. The news media prominently feature new health studies that range from the latest findings on diet to health care reform. In the fall of 2001, the media produced daily reports on anthrax-related attacks and other aspects of bioterrorism. Health news is routinely reported in television and radio broadcasts, newspapers, books, magazines, newsletters, Internet Web sites, and list servs. There are cable TV channels and network TV shows devoted primarily to health topics, and an estimated one-fourth of all daily newspaper articles are on health.[6]

Improvements in public health based on communicating information outside the scientific community can take a long time and may not always be successful, but there are many examples where it has made a difference. The 1964 Surgeon General's Report on Smoking and Health[7] and reports linking between aspirin use to Reye's syndrome are dramatic examples.[8] The long-term impact of communicating health messages can be profound, as evidenced by the decline in cigarette smoking from 1965 to 1990.[9] Communicating the adverse effects of tetraethyl lead to policy makers resulted in national legislation that eliminated automobiles running on leaded gasoline; [10] communicating about the benefits of folic acid help promoted fortification of bread with this compound.[11]

There are many success stories showing where effective communication has made a difference in the health of populations. Appropriate presentations of immunization research findings to policy makers, health care providers, and the public were critical in dramatically reducing the incidence of several infectious diseases.[12] Information about the effectiveness of mammography has been widely communicated to advocacy groups, policy makers, health care providers, and the general public, resulting in substantial increases in mammography screening.

Good communication of public health information may not be the primary reason for a major change in public policy or individual behavior; however, when public health practitioners do not communicate with nonscientific audiences or do so poorly, decisions will almost surely be based on other factors such as political pressure or economic incentive.[13]

BACKGROUND

With the exception of selected items reported in a few major journals (e.g., *New England Journal of Medicine, JAMA, Science*) or syntheses such as Reports of the U.S. Surgeon General or the National Academy of Sciences, findings intended for the scientific community are unlikely to be readily available to nonscientific audiences.[14] There are an estimated 25,000 scientific journals in the world;[15] the number of government-sponsored publications and scientific meetings is unknown but probably exceeds that of scientific journals by a substantial amount. Rarely does one study, report, or presentation to a scientific audience lead to immediate action—most simply add to the archive of scientific knowledge.

DEFINITIONS

Conceivably, the term public health could encompass any health issue that affects a member of the public. In this book, public health refers to the eight major areas that are typically the responsibility of federal, state, or local health departments in the United States: infectious disease; chronic disease; environmental and occupational health; health care services; mental health; injury; reproductive, maternal, and child health; and oral health.

The terms data and information are sometimes used interchangeably, but they have somewhat different meanings in this context. *Public health data* refer to numbers associated or applied to a given population, such as counts, rates, ratios, or percentages. *Public health information,* as used in this book, is a broader term that encompasses data but also includes interpretations and recommendations based on scientific knowledge. For example, reporting that there were 223,000 hospitalizations from pneumonia in the United States in 1997[16] is public health data; stating that "influenza vaccination reduces the risk of developing pneumonia among the elderly" is public health information.

AUDIENCES FOR PUBLIC HEALTH INFORMATION

Many people are potentially interested in public health information, but the level of interest varies greatly by topic and salience involvement. Hundreds of thousands of people may be interested when municipal water supplies are contaminated[17] or when research is released on the effects of day care on children's health,[18] but in some instances, only one person, perhaps the state health commissioner or a member of the general public, will have an interest.

In general, there are seven audiences for public health information: public health professionals; health care providers; patients (or consumers) in health care settings; the general public; the news media; policy makers (elected officials and administrators); and private or voluntary health organization members (Table 1.1). Communication with public health professionals, health care providers, and patients has been extensively described elsewhere.[19-20] This book focuses on communicating public health information to the general public, news media, policy makers, and individuals within private or voluntary organizations.

The majority of persons in these groups have not been educated in scientific disciplines or methods; the word nonscientist[21] is used throughout the book to describe persons not

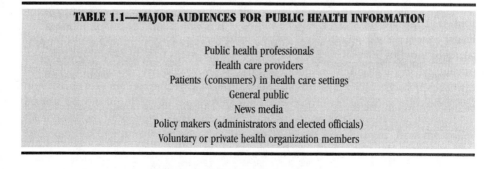

TABLE 1.1—MAJOR AUDIENCES FOR PUBLIC HEALTH INFORMATION

Public health professionals
Health care providers
Patients (consumers) in health care settings
General public
News media
Policy makers (administrators and elected officials)
Voluntary or private health organization members

working in scientific professions to whom public health professionals are trying to communicate public health information. Because of the lack of scientific training, it is essential to translate scientific concepts, terminology, and findings into more familiar terms in order to communicate them effectively. It is necessary to remember that the scientist/nonscientist dichotomy is somewhat artificial, as familiarity and understanding of science by individuals falls along a continuum. Also, there can be overlap between groups: an administrator may also be a health care practitioner and voluntary health organizations may employ established scientists.

Each nonscientific audience has its own distinctive characteristics. General public audiences rarely consist of everyone; instead, they are usually segmented (stratified) by certain characteristics such as demographics or lifestyle patterns.[22] The news media consists of persons in television, radio, Internet, magazines and newspapers, and plays a critical role in communicating information and influencing all the other audiences.[6,23]

Policy makers include administrators and elected officials who have the authority to make decisions about laws, regulations, other policies, programs, and resources that affect many people. Examples of policy makers include heads of public health agencies, city council members, state legislators, and federal legislators. The many private health and voluntary organizations potentially interested in public health information include advocacy groups, professional associations, and voluntary associations such as the American Cancer Society. (Each of the nonscientific audiences is discussed in detail in chapters 4 through 8.)

BARRIERS TO COMMUNICATION

LACK OF INTEREST OR LOW PRIORITY

Public health professionals have many roles and duties; their responsibilities depend on their profession, training, and work setting. Some practitioners do not like communicating with nonscientific audiences and make it a low priority. It takes some extra effort, for example, to translate public health research findings into simpler words that can be understood by the lay public. Audiences members may also challenge the assumptions and interpretations behind public health knowledge, and can make practitioners feel uncomfortable.

Examples from academic institutions and state health departments are revealing in this regard. Most academics' duties consist of teaching students and conducting research that leads to publication in scientific journals. They seldom interact with nonscientists, and are generally rewarded based on successful "grantsmanship" and a record of publications. When research performed by academics is communicated outside the scientific community, it is often a result of their institution's efforts (e.g., a public relations officer) or by staff representing the scientific journals. There may even be negative peer pressure not to interact with the lay public, as scientists who communicate directly with advocacy groups or with the media may be viewed by other scientists as unprofessional or self-promoting.[6,24] State health department employees are more likely than academics to routinely communicate with nonscientists, especially with representatives of organizations or the general public. These public health practitioners are usually involved in program activities, planning, administration, and technical assistance. However, much of their communication is with others involved in the health field. Written communication may occur through routine state reports or publications, but such products are often not timely and are targeted for the public health community. Although state health departments often employ communication specialists, public health practitioners in state government are usually discouraged from interacting with certain nonscientific audiences, such as news media, for fear of providing mixed messages or political embarrassment.

Despite the lack of interest and low priority for communication, public health professionals who take the time to communicate with nonscientific audiences usually find it to be a positive experience. For example, in a study of scientists who had articles published in *JAMA* and the *New England Journal of Medicine*, a total of 86% of authors reported that media coverage of their stories was accurate and 84% believed that the coverage benefited the general public.[24]

BELIEF THAT DATA SPEAK FOR THEMSELVES

Another barrier is the mistaken belief that data speak for themselves. Math literacy and math interest in the United States is low;[25] many people do not understand fractions, rates, odds ratios, or percentages, all of which are commonly used in public health reporting. Scientific methods and reasoning are unfamiliar to many people; instead, they often rely on personal experience, stories, and emotion to make health decisions.[26] Legal and legislative hearings provide ample evidence of this, as anecdotes and nonverbal communication are usually more persuasive than data presentations. It is not just the general public that has trouble with numbers: many news media representatives and policy makers are also not mathematically inclined and may distrust numbers.[25,27]

The implication of low math literacy and interest is that most people will not be persuaded solely by logical, number-driven arguments: presenting more data and facts to such audiences is likely to be counterproductive. This does not mean that public health professionals should not use quantitative information; it does mean that such information needs to be translated into a form appropriate for the intended audience (chapter 3).[6]

LACK OF KNOWLEDGE ON HOW TO COMMUNICATE

Finally and perhaps most importantly, many practitioners do not know how to communicate public health information well. Such skills can be learned, but they are rarely taught in professional schools or continuing education courses.[6] This is in marked contrast to other fields such as business, where training in communication, especially in understanding the interests of an audience, is highly emphasized.[28]

Most public health professionals do not fully understand the background, interests, and needs of nonscientific audiences. An illustrative example concerns communicating with the news media. With few exceptions, newspaper, radio, and television reporters operate on very short deadlines and need rapid responses to interview requests (chapter 6). Indeed, some media representatives sensationalize health stories, but most reporters are simply asking for information from public health professionals and interactions are rarely confrontational. Reporters generally are looking for the "bottom line", that is, what the findings are, what they mean, and how best to proceed. If public health professionals understand news reporters' motivations better, they are likely to have frequent (and positive) encounters with media representatives, thereby helping to facilitate the spread of public health information to a broad audience.

THE FIELD OF HEALTH COMMUNICATION

DESCRIPTION

Health communication has been defined as "the study and use of methods to inform and influence individual and community decisions that enhance health."[29] It is a hybrid discipline that draws primarily from 8 areas: 1) communication; 2) behavioral science; 3) health education and health promotion; 4) journalism; 5) business; 6) health professions (e.g., medicine, nursing); 7) political science; and 8) information technology. Consistent with their varied backgrounds, health communication specialists focus on areas ranging from patient-provider interactions to mass communication campaigns.

Communication has existed for more than 50 years as a unique discipline and has provided a large body of scientific research on interpersonal, group, and mass communication. Most major universities have faculty and degree programs in this area. The increased knowledge of human behavior gained from research in psychology, sociology, demography, and anthropology has been extensively applied to health communication, especially through the disciplines of health education and health promotion.[30,31] Communication strategies and approaches are commonly based on theories derived from behavioral science such as health belief, self-efficacy, and trans-theoretical models[32] (see chapters 4 and 5).

Health journalists have played a key role translating health information to nonscientific audiences through print, radio, and television. Major newspapers and magazines have health writers, and there are many health-specific journals designed for lay audiences.[6] Best-selling nonfiction and fiction books have covered public health topics such as environmental degradation,[33] physical fitness,[34] and infectious disease outbreaks.[35] Television networks and cable channels often employ health reporters, and, increasingly, health communication experts provide public health messages to the mass entertainment industry (e.g., through television and movie story lines).[36]

Health communication also draws heavily from experience and research in business, especially marketing and advertising;[22,30] one example of this is the use of social marketing in public health promotion.[22,30] A major contribution from business theory has been audience segmentation, or targeting health messages to specific audiences.[22,30] Health professions represent another broad area that has contributed to health communication. This has been especially true for communication in clinical settings, with nursing involved perhaps more often than other health professions.[26]

Political science, especially advocacy, also contributes to health communication. This is most evident in the area of media advocacy, which is the attempt to use the news media to influence public health policy.[23,37] Finally, a recent contributor to the field has been the area of information technology, or informatics.[38] Advances in information science, engineering, and computer technology have provided new opportunities to communicate health information, such as electronic mail and Internet web sites.

Some aspects of health communication have a long history. Public health campaigns, (e.g., smallpox inoculation and temperance) have occurred in the United States since the 1700s.[39,40] Such campaigns have typically been led by strong-willed individual advocates who used newspaper articles, pamphlets, and legislative testimony to galvanize broad interest and action. So-called muckraking journalists in the late 1890s and early 1900s stressed public health issues such as unsafe food and child labor. Voluntary organizations became involved in health communication efforts starting in the late 1800s; by the 1920s, the American Cancer Society had developed a message about cancer warning signs for the public.[40]

ROLE FOR PUBLIC HEALTH PRACTICE

Knowledge and implementation of health communication principles can greatly enhance the practice of public health. Fundamentally, health communication emphasizes the importance of communicating (why), the audience, and the message to be communicated, and it stresses the need for a plan of action.[41] Public health professionals must understand their audiences and the environments in which they operate; this is a key tenet of successful health communication.

The importance of communication as a critical skill for public health practice is increasingly being recognized. A major step forward in this recognition came in the spring of 2001, when the Council on Linkages Between Academia and Public Health Practice adopted a set of core competencies for practitioners.[42] (Partners and sponsors of the Council included organizations and agencies such as the Association of Schools of Public Health, American Public Health Association, Association of State and Territorial Health Officials, Centers for Disease Control and Prevention, National Association of County and City Health Officials, National Library of Medicine, Society of Public Health Education, American College of Preventive Medicine, and the Public Health Foundation.[42]) The anthrax attacks in 2001[43] provided even further evidence of the importance of communication for public health.

The competencies adopted by the Council were divided into eight domains—Domain number 3 is Communication Skills (Table 1.2). This book covers 4 of the 6 specific communication skills competencies recommended by the Council: written and oral communication; advocacy for public health programs and resources; use of advanced technology and community networks; and accurate presentation of demographic, statistical, programmatic, and other information to different audiences.

Understanding and applying health communication principles requires time and experience, and practitioners should obtain guidance whenever possible from persons with this specialized expertise. Examples of such persons include graphic or visual artists, public relations or press (media) officers, Internet Web site designers, risk communication experts,

---

TABLE 1.2—RECOMMENDED CORE COMPETENCY COMMUNICATION SKILLS FOR PUBLIC HEALTH PROFESSIONALS

1. Communicates effectively both in writing and orally, or in other ways
2. Solicits input from individuals and organizations
3. Advocates for public health programs and resources
4. Leads and participates in groups to address specific issues
5. Uses the media, advanced technologies, and community networks to communicate information
6. Effectively presents accurate demographic, statistical, programmatic, and scientific information for professional and lay audiences

Source: *Council on Linkages Between Academia and Public Health Practice (Reference 42)*

and experts in writing for low literacy audiences. Multidisciplinary teams are often essential to maximize the effectiveness of communication activities, especially for larger efforts such as programs targeting mass audiences.

SUMMARY

Communicating health information outside the health community is an important role for practitioners. The nonscientific audiences that are the focus of this book include the general public, news media, policy makers, and members of private or voluntary health organizations.

Communication with nonscientific audiences is often limited in scope or execution because practitioners do not make it a priority, they believe that data speak for themselves, and they may not know how to communicate effectively. Public health professionals can learn from the field of health communication how to understand and meet the communication needs of nonscientific audiences.

Many practitioners recognize the need to develop and improve their communication skills. The Council on Linkages Between Academia and Public Health Practice has adopted communication as a core competency for practitioners. In this information age, it is likely that the paradigm for public health will continue to shift to one that increasingly stresses information synthesis and presentation. [44]

CHAPTER 1 ENDNOTES

1. Wynder EL. Applied epidemiology. *Am J Epidemiol.* 1985;121:781-82.
2. Siegel M, Doner L. *Marketing Public Health: Strategies to Promote Social Change.* Gaithersburg, MD: Aspen; 1998.
3. Centers for Disease Control and Prevention. Update: multistate outbreak of Escherichia coli O157:H7 infections from hamburgers—western United States, 1992-1993. *MMWR.* 1993;42:258-263.
4. Peterson DE, Zeger SL, Remington PL, Anderson HA. The effect of state cigarette excise taxes on cigarette sales, 1955 to 1988. *Am J Public Health.* 1992;82:94-96.
5. Kulldorff M, Feuer EJ, Miller BA, Freedman LS. Breast cancer clusters in the northeast United States: a geographic analysis. *Am J Epidemiol.* 1997;146:161-170.
6. Atkin C, Wallack L, eds. *Mass Communication and Public Health: Complexities and Conflicts.* Newbury Park, CA: Sage; 1990.
7. U.S. Department of Health, Education, and Welfare. U.S. Public Health Service. *Smoking and Health. Report of the Advisory Committee to the Surgeon General of the Public Health Service.* Washington, DC: Center for Disease Control; Publication (PHS) 11-3; 1964.
8. Hurwitz ES. Reye's syndrome. *Epidemiol Rev.* 1989;11:249-253.
9. Giovino GA, Schooley MW, Zhu BP, et al. Surveillance for selected tobacco-use behaviors—United States, 1990-1994. *MMWR CDC Surveillance Summaries.* 1994;43:1-43.
10. Annest JL, Pirkle JL, Makuc D, Neese JW, Bayse DD, Kovar MG. Chronological trends in blood lead levels between 1976 and 1980. *N Engl J Med.* 1983;308:1373-77.
11. Czeik AE, Dudas J. Prevention of first occurrence of neural tube defects by periconceptional vitamin supplementation. *N Engl J Med.* 1992;327:1832-1835.
12. Centers for Disease Control and Prevention. Achievements in public health, 1900-1999: impact of vaccines universally recommended for children—United States, 1900-1998. *MMWR.* 1999;48:243-248.
13. Crossen C. *Tainted Truth: The Manipulation of Fact in America.* New York: Simon & Schuster; 1994.
14. deSemir V, Ribas C, Reveulta G. Press releases of science journal articles and subsequent newspaper stories on the same topic. *JAMA.* 1998;280:294-295.
15. Johnson T. Shattuck lecture—medicine and the media. *N Eng J Med.* 1998;339:87-92.
16. National Center for Health Statistics. *Health, United States, 2000 with Adolescent Health Chartbook.*

Hyattsville, MD: National Center for Health Statistics; 2000.

17. MacKenzie WR, Hoxie JJ, Proctor ME, et al. A massive outbreak in Milwaukee of cryptosporidium infection transmitted through the public water supply. *N Engl J Med.* 1994;331:161-167.

18. Zoritch B, Roberts I, Oakley A. Day care for pre-school children. *Cochrane Database Syst Rev.* 2000;2:CD000564.

19. British Medical Association. *How to Do It.* London, England: British Medical Journal, 1985.

20. Hinz C. *Communicating with Your Patients: Skills for Building Rapport.* Chicago, IL: American Medical Association; 1999.

21. Friedman SM, Dunwoody S, Rogers CL, eds. *Scientists and Journalists: Reporting Science as News.* Washington, DC: American Association for the Advancement of Science, 1986.

22. Andreasen AR. *Marketing Social Change.* San Francisco: Jossey-Bass; 1995.

23. Wallack L, Dorfman L, Jernigan D, Themba M. *Media Advocacy and Public Health.* Newbury Park, CA: Sage; 1993.

24. Wilkes MS, Kravitz RL. Medical researchers and the media: attitudes toward public dissemination of research. *JAMA.* 1992;268:999-1003.

25. Paulos JA. *Innumeracy: Mathematical Illiteracy and its Consequences.* New York: Farrar, Straus, & Giroux; 1989.

26. Northouse LL, Northouse PG. *Health Communication: Strategies for Health Professionals.* 3rd ed. Stamford, CT: Appleton & Lange; 1998.

27. Huff D. *How to Lie with Statistics.* 38th ed. New York: WW Norton & Company; 1982.

28. Spendolini MJ. *The Benchmarking Book.* New York: Amacom, 1992.

29. Freimuth V, Cole G, Kirby S. Issues in evaluating mass mediated health communication campaigns. In: Rootman I, Goodstadt M, Hyndman B, et al, eds. *Evaluation in Health Promotion: Principles and Perspectives.* Geneva: WHO Regional Publications, European Series, No. 92, 2001.

30. Kotler P, Roberto EL. *Social Marketing: Strategies for Changing Public Behavior.* New York: The Free Press; 1989.

31. Maibach E, Parrott RL, eds. *Designing Health Messages: Approaches from Communication Theory and Public Health Practice.* Thousand Oaks, CA: Sage; 1995.

32. National Cancer Institute. *Theory at a Glance: A Guide for Health Promotion Practice.* Bethesda, MD: National Cancer Institute; 1995. NIH Pub. No. 95-3896.

33. Carson R. *Silent Spring.* Boston: Houghton Mifflin; 1962.

34. Cooper KH. *The New Aerobics.* New York: Bantam Books; 1970.

35. Crichton M. *The Andromeda Strain.* New York: Knopf; 1969.

36. Montgomery KC. Promoting health through entertainment television. In: Atkin C, Wallack L, eds. *Mass Communication and Public Health.* Newbury Park, CA: Sage; 1990.

37. Wallack L, Woodruff K, Dorfman L, Diaz I. *News for a Change: An Advocate's Guide to Working with the Media.* Thousand Oaks, CA: Sage; 1999.

38. Kilbourne EM. Informatics in public health surveillance: current issues and future perspectives. In: Wetterhall SF, ed. Proceedings of the 1992 International Symposium on Public Health Surveillance. *MMWR.* 1992 (suppl);41:91-99.

39. Behr E. *Prohibition: Thirteen Years that Changed America.* New York: Arcade Publishing; 1996.

40. Paisley W. Public health communications campaigns: the American experiences. In: Rice RE, Atkin CK, eds. *Public Communication Campaigns.* 3rd ed. Thousand Oaks, CA: Sage; 2001:3-21.

41. McGuire WJ. Theoretical foundations of campaigns. In: Rice RE, Atkin CK, eds. *Public Communication Campaigns.* 2nd ed. Newbury Park, CA: Sage Publications; 1989:43-65.

42. Council on Linkages Between Academia and Public Health Practice. *Consensus Set of Core Competencies.* Washington, DC: Public Health Foundation, 2001. Available at: http://trainingfinder.org/competencies. Date accessed: March 5, 2002.

43. Borio L, Frank D, Mani V, et al. Death due to bioterrorism-related inhalational anthrax: report of 2 patients. *JAMA.* 2001;28:2554-9.

44. Brownson RC, Kreuter MW. Future trends affecting public health: challenges and opportunities. *J Public Health Management Practice.* 1997;3:49-60.

SUGGESTED READINGS AND RESOURCES

Atkin C, Wallack L, eds. *Mass Communication and Public Health: Complexities and Conflicts.* Newbury Park, CA: Sage; 1990.

Council on Linkages Between Academia and Public Health Practice. *Consensus Set of Core Competencies.* Washington, DC: Public Health Foundation, 2001. Available at: http://trainingfinder.org/competencies.

Maibach E, Parrott RL, eds. *Designing Health Messages: Approaches from Communication Theory and Public Health Practice.* Thousand Oaks, CA: Sage; 1995.

Remington PL. Communicating epidemiologic information. In: Brownson RC, Petitti DB, eds. *Applied Epidemiology: Theory to Practice.* New York: Oxford University Press; 1998:323-348.

Siegel M, Doner L. *Marketing Public Health: Strategies to Promote Social Change.* Gaithersburg, MD: Aspen; 1998.

Chapter Two

PUBLIC HEALTH COMMUNICATION: A PLANNING FRAMEWORK

Claudia Parvanta, PhD
Edward Maibach, PhD
Elaine Arkin
David E. Nelson MD, MPH
Jennifer Woodward, PhD

C hapter 1 describes some of the reasons why the public appears to be more interested in health today, as well as some of the challenges in communicating health information to nonscientific audiences. Communication between public health practitioners and nonscientific audiences occurs on many levels. These can include encouraging the public to increase physical activity, informing public and policy makers about environmental or infectious disease emergencies such as food-borne outbreaks, advocating to administrators for program resources, and encouraging elected officials to enact new policies that enhance the public's health such as lowering the legal blood alcohol level for automobile drivers.

As different as these communication tasks are in their urgency and focus, they can all be managed by following a basic planning framework. This chapter presents an overview of the public health communication framework used throughout this book, and provides five examples of applying the framework to situations common in public health practice.

BACKGROUND

In public health, communication can play either a supporting or a lead role. At times it is used primarily to provide information, for example, raising awareness about a new or urgent health problem (e.g., disease outbreak or natural disaster), or informing policy makers or the public about research findings and health trends. At other times, persuasive communication is used to encourage changes in public attitudes or health behaviors, reduce fear, or influence support for public health programs or policies. Public health communication—particularly behavior change communication—is based on a platform of scientific evidence arising from research studies and surveillance data. Before launching into any communication activity, it is important to consider the role that health information or persuasive communication can play in relation to policies, programs, or structural changes that affect the public's health.

While communication is only part of the picture, it can be quite powerful. All communication is based on achieving certain results when a sender (source) transmits a message to a receiver. The Hierarchy of Effects Model[1] suggests that the way a message is created and transmitted affects, in this order, whether the recipient: (1) is exposed to the message, (2) pays attention, (3) is interested, (4) understands, (5) learns a skill, (6) changes an attitude, (7) retains the information (short duration), (8) can recall the information (long duration), (9) makes a decision, (10) performs an action, (11) reinforces the action, and (12) organizes other life experience to maintain the action indefinitely. While the Hierarchy of Effects Model has been revised over the years, nearly all communication planning involves acquiring the necessary information to shape what goes into a communication experience so that one or more of these effects will result, and an evaluation to measure whether these effects took place.[2]

As might be expected, experience and research have demonstrated that more effort is required to achieve the higher levels of effect in the hierarchy. But many health communication programs fail because they do not even reach the first step—creating exposure—let alone aiding a decision or prompting action. Neither the most accurate data or the most poignant stories can inform or persuade anyone if they are not seen or heard.

The framework described in this chapter is based on best practices in public health communication, and is consistent with the approach recommended by federal agencies such as the Centers for Disease Control and Prevention (CDC), the National Institutes of Health, and the United States Agency for International Development (USAID).[3,4] It is designed to aid public health practitioners achieve communication goals consistent with the Hierarchy of Effects Model, such as gaining the attention of an audience, informing them, or persuading them to take action.

The framework is versatile and can be applied in most public health communication situations. It can be used both in reactive communication situations, such as when an audience requests information from a practitioner, and in proactive communication situations where practitioners seek to gain the attention and interest of the audience. The communication framework can be applied when communicating with mass audiences or with individual policy makers.

PUBLIC HEALTH COMMUNICATION FRAMEWORK

Public health communication planning consists of 8 interrelated steps: (1) Assessing the science; (2) Defining the purpose for the communication; (3) Identifying the audience(s) and understanding their characteristics; (4) Developing and testing message concepts; (5) Choosing media and channels for the message; (6) Determining the best timing for delivering the message; (7) Implementing the communication plan; and (8) Evaluating the effort and its impact (Table 2.1). This can be thought of as finding answers to the following questions:

- What is the scientific evidence?
- Why is communication necessary?
- Who is the audience?

TABLE 2.1—PUBLIC HEALTH COMMUNICATION PLANNING FRAMEWORK		
Sequence	**Planning Step**	**Question to be Answered**
1	Assess the science	What is the scientific evidence?
2	Define the purpose: Inform or Persuade	Why is communication necessary?
3	Identify the audience(s) and understand their characteristics	Who is the audience?
4	Develop and test message concepts	What is the message?
5	Choose media and channels	How and where should the message be delivered?
6	Determine timing	When should the message be disseminated?
7	Implement the Communication Plan	
8	Evaluate the effort and its impact	Did the audience receive the information and was it effective?

- What is the message?
- How and where should the message be delivered?
- When should the message be delivered?
- Was the communication effective?

Choosing media and channels for the message, determining the timing, and evaluating the effort and its impact (steps 5, 6 and 8) will not be included in every communication effort. However, assessing the science, defining the purpose, and identifying and understanding the audience (steps 1 through 3) will determine the message and the tactical communication plan (steps 5-6) and must be part of every health communication planning effort. Each of the steps in the planning framework is discussed in more detail in the pages that follow.

STEP 1: ASSESS THE SCIENCE

The basis for responsible public health communication is scientific knowledge and consensus. Most health-promoting activities or interventions are initiated once sufficient scientific evidence exists on the value of individual behavior change or the value of the societal or structural changes necessary to facilitate adoption of healthy behaviors or other interventions.[5] Public health practitioners may need to weigh the scientific evidence themselves; in many situations findings are contradictory, unclear, or potentially flawed. Practitioners have a responsibility to examine the quality of the available scientific information prior to performing any communication activity.

In addition to assessing the science, practitioners also need to be able to explain the science in terms understandable to nonscientific audiences. Public opinion polls suggest that large public health agencies are considered credible,[6] but that this trust can be easily lost.[7] As Christine Russell, Special Health Correspondent to the Washington Post suggested, "Scientists need to put as much emphasis on explaining their study to the public as in getting it published in the right journal. Clinicians need to understand the larger picture to help put a given risk in context when patients call. Journalists need to be better equipped to ask the right questions and interpret the answers . . ."[8] Failure to play an active part in the interpretation of scientific findings can be damaging to the public, the communicator, and the field of public health. (Assessing the science and translating data to nonscientific audiences is covered in chapter 3.)

STEP 2: DEFINE THE PURPOSE FOR THE COMMUNICATION

The purpose of communication is always audience-specific, and it must target what the recipient is meant to do in response to the message. Public health practitioners often first encounter a situation where communication is necessary; how to target specific audiences is the next consideration.

Overall Purpose: To Inform or to Persuade? In this book, informing means providing factual information with no intent of influencing a decision. Individuals and policy makers need information to make decisions, and much of the information gathered by public health practitioners is devoted to this end. Even when a public health practitioner is "just providing numbers," someone at some point in time thought these numbers were necessary for making a decision. Thus, even the most mundane statistical report should be viewed with an eye to facilitating decision-making. Theories and techniques to enhance the information value of health communication for the public are discussed in chapter 4.

Beyond informing, many public health practitioners hope that their communications persuade individuals to change their health behavior or result in the creation of policies, programs, or laws that support healthy living. Techniques to influence or persuade audiences must often provide additional social and cultural information (e.g., expert opinion; testimonials; references to persons, places, values or things that are meaningful to a particular individual or group of people). Persuasive communication also relies on theories about how individuals or groups make decisions to change behavior; these theories are discussed in chapter 5.

Choosing to inform or persuade audiences is a decision with ethical dimensions. [9,10] In public health, ethics are largely determined by the scientific consensus about the issue in question and by the intended and unintended outcomes of interventions for all persons. When there is consensus about the beneficial value of a given health behavior for the individual and for society, it is considered ethical to attempt to persuade individuals to adopt that behavior (e.g., not using tobacco, being physically active), or to persuade policy makers to enact policies, support programs, or provide resources to improve health (e.g., mandatory immunization laws for school-age children). Failing to advocate for such individual and social changes when the scientific evidence is strong has ethical dilemmas of its own.[5,11]

When scientific consensus does not exist on a specific topic, when there are potentially serious side-effects involved, or when personal values are critical to a decision, it may be more appropriate simply to present the information but allow individuals to make informed decisions on their own. Expansion of genetic testing or the use of hormone replacement therapy in post-menopausal women are current examples.

The difference between informing and persuading may be difficult to discern, and some argue that all health communication is persuasive.[12] Informational and persuasive messages are commonly used concurrently (e.g., "the number of uninsured persons is increasing and here's what needs to be done to reduce this problem"). Beyond informing and persuading, specific communication objectives need to be developed depending on how far up the Hierarchy of Effects scale practitioners or programs plan to go in their communication efforts.[1]

STEP 3: IDENTIFY THE AUDIENCES AND UNDERSTAND THEIR CHARACTERISTICS

A fundamental tenet of health communication is to identify and understand the intended audience. While identifying the audience is straightforward in the case of communicating with an individual administrator, elected official, or member of the public, some effort is still necessary to understand these individuals' backgrounds or their interest in a topic. Identifying and understanding larger general public audiences is especially challenging; even when "everyone" needs to know something, rarely can all people understand or relate to the same messages or make effective use of the same communication media.

Audience segmentation is the process of dividing people (usually the general public) into relatively homogenous groups for the purpose of communicating information. The members of these audience "segments" need to be similar enough to each other and distinct enough from other groups along dimensions that are meaningful to the health communication effort.[5] There are practical reasons for doing audience segmentation,[13-16] including more efficient use of program time and financial resources. Audience segmentation is the basis for communication planning, including developing a rationale for message content, making tactical decisions about the communications (format), selecting the real or "virtual" location (channel) where the audience will encounter the message, and the schedule required to reach as much of the intended audience as often as considered necessary.

Many of the most successful communication efforts segment audiences by one or more of the following 4 categories:

1. As individuals or policy makers
2. By demographic, cultural, and other personal characteristics
3. By psychological factors (e.g., interest in an issue, or readiness to adopt a new behavior; these are referred to as "involvement level" or "readiness stage" in the health communication literature)
4. By the relationship of one group or individual to another in terms of ability to influence or share information (primary, secondary, or tertiary audiences)

Individuals and policy makers Is the intended beneficiary of the information using it for a personal decision or one affecting the welfare of others? Dividing the audience into individuals or policy makers is a fairly crude but important distinction. Both of these audiences require more specific characterization; for example, policy makers might be local elected officials, heads of government agencies, or high-level administrators for a health care organization. Their interest in specific issues will vary, and they are not identical in how they perceive and use information.

The audience and the purpose for communicating are closely interrelated (Table 2.2). The need to collect additional information about audience characteristics will be largely determined by examining the purpose of the communication (informing vs. persuading) and whether it will be directed to individuals trying to make decisions for their own welfare or to policy makers trying to make decisions that effect broader audiences. Persuasive approaches require that messages and communication media be more closely matched to the characteristics of the audience than informational messages, especially when trying to reach individuals.

Demographic, cultural, and other personal characteristics Health behavior concepts and materials often need to be customized or tailored to suit the target audience. Collecting information about the demographics, cultural identity, information processing abilities, and other personal characteristics of the intended audience is essential to this task. Communicating about sexual issues or domestic violence issues, for example, depends heavily on factors such as the age, gender, educational level, and cultural background of the intended audience. Other important considerations include language comprehension and literacy. These issues are discussed at some length in chapter 4.

Psychological factors Segmentation strategies become more strategic at this level, focusing on psychological factors such as interest in an issue, readiness to change a behavior, or sense of ability to make a change (self-efficacy).[17] Level of interest (involvement) may play an overriding role in determining whether diverse audiences pay attention to messages.[13] For example, women hoping to become pregnant within the next year have a high level of involvement in pregnancy and childbirth issues compared to women who are not planning to become pregnant; different messages are necessary to reach each of these audiences.[18] For large-scale health communication campaigns, in-depth research is often necessary to categorize audiences based on involvement level.

Level of involvement also affects communication with policy makers. Policy makers are concerned about issues that affect their constituency and for which they believe they are responsible or will be held accountable. Determining the level of concern among constituency groups or relevant stakeholders is very helpful to assess the involvement level of policy makers. If these constituency groups are highly involved, communicators can report to policy makers about the interest and support of these key audiences, provide potential solutions, and indicate how policy makers can take a positive ("champion") role on issues.

TABLE 2.2—GENERAL RELATIONSHIP BETWEEN THE PURPOSE AND THE AUDIENCE IN PUBLIC HEALTH COMMUNICATION

Purpose (Why)	Audience (Who)	
	Individuals	*Policy Makers*
Inform	Examples Increase knowledge Facilitate informed decision making	Examples Increase knowledge Facilitate informed decision making
Persuade	Examples Change attitude or behavior Learn new skill	Examples Change or maintain program, policy or law Change or maintain resources

Related to level of involvement is readiness stage. This is based on the Transtheoretical (or Stages-of-Change) Model[19] (chapter 5). This model can be used to identify smaller groups within an otherwise homogenous audience based on their readiness to adopt new behaviors.[20] Sometimes the readiness stage supercedes other audience characteristics; for example, people who have tried to quit smoking previously or who are in an active process of quitting.

Primary, secondary, and tertiary audiences The final audience consideration is the relationship of one group or individual to others in terms of their ability to share information or influence decisions. The health communication term for this is primary, secondary, and tertiary audiences.[4] As implied by the rank order, primary audiences consist of those persons who need to make a decision or a change. The secondary audience normally includes persons in a position to directly influence the decisions or actions of the primary audience. For individuals, examples include family or peer group members, teachers, or physicians; for policy makers, this would include important stakeholders or the news media. Tertiary audiences generally are the farthest away from individuals making decisions about individual health activities or policies, but they can still play an important role in shaping social norms or professional values. Examples of tertiary audiences include health care professional associations, religious organizations, and community leaders.

Depending on the situation, targeting communication efforts toward secondary or tertiary audiences can be effective. For example, efforts to improve receipt of clinical preventive services such as adult immunization will be enhanced if communication efforts target health care providers as the secondary audience. Similarly, efforts to encourage elected officials to enact legislation may be enhanced by targeting communication efforts toward private or voluntary health organizations.

In summary, whether trying to reach a specific individual or a large population group, identifying and understanding audiences is a crucial yet often overlooked step in public health communication. To do this well requires a commitment to researching audience characteristics prior to message development (see discussions on formative research later in this chapter). For large-scale health communication campaigns directed towards the general public, much information about target audiences can be obtained from existing databases; for example, both CDC and NIH make use of the PRIZM© system offered by Claritas[7], as well as other marketing data bases created for special populations such as youth or Hispanic populations. For large-scale campaigns, analyses of databases such as these should precede in-depth qualitative research to gain a more complete understanding of the intended audience groups.

STEP 4: DEVELOP AND TEST MESSAGE CONCEPTS

Message development involves condensing and translating scientific information into simple and readily understood words and visual images. The message and its delivery must first create attention and interest before it can inform or persuade audiences.

The type of message greatly depends on the communication purpose (i.e., to inform or persuade) and the audience. When informing audiences, it is essential to focus on the most important information and state this clearly and succinctly. The journalistic concept of the "single overriding health communication objective," or SOHCO, is used to condense complex scientific information into a few key statements (chapter 6). The SOHCO is applicable to all audiences, not only the news media, as it can help prevent important information from getting lost in a sea of details.

Developing persuasive messages begins with this same approach of identifying the key pieces of information, but practitioners also must consider psychological and other factors that influence how audiences receive the information. Often what practitioners believe to be a message is really an optimal health behavior (e.g., eat five servings of fruits or vegetables daily) or descriptions about what to do, where to go, or when to act in a particular situation. Such messages are often not very persuasive because the information is easily ignored. To make a message more compelling, it should use words, body language, tone of voice, imagery, and other communication features that appeal to specific audiences.

When working with multicultural audiences, attention must be paid to how different groups perceive the verbiage and other features of a message. Many cultures prefer to use metaphors, proverbs, stories, or songs to convey complex information indirectly. Western-style factual statements, particularly when used in a persuasive situation, are sometimes rejected for being too cold, too direct, or otherwise in conflict with more traditional beliefs, values, and ways of seeking communication and receiving health care.[21,22]

Identifying potential audiences and pretesting messages is a critical component of message development and delivery, especially for persuasive communication, and is called formative evaluation.[4] It consists of testing messages with persons familiar with the subject (often professional colleagues) and testing messages with intended audiences. The extent to which pretesting is done depends on timing, feasibility, and resources. Pretesting is often impractical in crisis situations, and may be difficult to do with policy makers because of their limited number and special status. Pretesting of messages is often done with surrogates for policy makers (e.g., their staff members), and their opinions can be invaluable for strong message development.

Despite the obstacles, every effort must be made to pretest messages and materials intended for mass media dissemination. A first level check of the message with colleagues helps to insure that message content is correct, but this says nothing about whether the intended audience will understand the messages. Qualitative methods such as focus groups or shopping mall intercept interviews are quick, efficient ways to pretest message concepts and finished materials. For larger public communication campaigns, more extensive quantitative methods, such as web-enabled panels that employ larger samples of individuals, can be used.

When resources and time are in short supply, rapid pretesting with individuals from organizations that serve the intended audience can increase message effectiveness.[11] While informal pretesting of messages with friends or relatives provides a basic measure of comprehension by target audiences, it is not recommended unless the communication activity is given a very low priority. Table 2.3 lists the elements and considerations for pretesting messages with general public audiences; further discussion on testing messages with the general public is covered in chapter 4.

STEP 5: CHOOSE THE MEDIA AND CHANNELS FOR THE MESSAGE

Function often dictates form when considering the medium (format) and dissemination channels (outlets) for messages. For example, consider the Internet, music video tel-

TABLE 2.3—SUGGESTED ITEMS TO COVER WHEN PRETESTING MESSAGES AND MATERIALS

Comprehension	Is the message clearly understood?
	Is the audience able to identify and recall the intended main messages?
	Is the intended information presented in a manner that makes it effective and actionable for the intended audience?
Liking	How much does the audience like the presentation?
	What elements do they especially like or dislike?
Personal Relevance	Do respondents perceive the messages as relevant to themselves personally as well as to their peers?
	Is the message consistent with their own perceptions and experience?
Believability	Is the message and/or its source perceived as credible?
	Does it portray the message realistically and convincingly?
Acceptability	Is there anything in the message that is perceived as offensive or unacceptable to either the primary or secondary audiences?
	Do parents have significant concerns about ads intended for youth audiences?
Behavioral Intent	Do respondents think they will take action as a result of seeing or hearing the message?

evision stations, and health care provider waiting rooms. The context in which the intended audience will encounter messages prescribes the way messages need to be produced. This can vary widely: how to deliver a message to a policy maker is vastly different than planning a mass media campaign directed towards teenagers, and will influence such things as choice of color, music, tone, spokesperson, text, etc. For this reason, communication media production and placement issues are considered together in this section.

Many health communication programs directed toward the general public, for example, begin with someone saying, "we need a brochure" or "we need a video." But as this framework suggests, the form of the communication media will be determined by decisions made during previous steps. Chapters 9–12 discuss issues of communicating health information through different media.

A communication channel is the vehicle that transmits a message from a source to a receiver.[23] Table 2.4 categorizes channels into four broad groups: interpersonal (or face-to-face) contact, written materials and audiovisuals, mass media, and electronic and other evolving media. The distinction between these channels has become somewhat blurred in recent years because of advances in information technology. For example, e-mail is most commonly used for exchanging information with one or few other users (interpersonal contact), but it also can be used to reach larger audiences that may be unknown to the sender. The development of tailored communication[24,25] allows messages and interactions to be personalized to individuals within larger audiences (e.g., through Internet Web sites, CD-ROM, automated phone messaging). Communicating with the news media to reach

TABLE 2.4 – COMMUNICATION CHANNELS AND EXAMPLES

Channel	Examples
Interpersonal contact	Face-to-face meetings (one-on-one or small groups), telephone conversations, patient-provider visits, public speaking, staffed mall kiosks
Written materials and audiovisuals	Correspondence, posters, brochures, fact sheets, 35 mm or Powerpoint© slides, videotapes, audiotapes
Mass Media	Movies, television, radio, newspapers, magazines, billboards
Electronic and other new media	Fax, CD-ROM, DVD, automatic voice messaging, e-mail, Internet Web sites, teleconferencing, videoconferencing

broader audiences, and certain aspects of electronic communication, are covered in chapters 6 and 12. Detailed discussions of other channels is beyond the scope of this book.

STEP 6: DETERMINE THE BEST TIMING FOR DELIVERING THE MESSAGE

When to communicate public health information is often straightforward, especially in reactive situations when there is a deadline. Such situations include notifying persons potentially at risk in acute outbreaks, toxic exposures, or disasters, when there is a clear health risk or danger.[26] Timing can also be critical in creating interest for an issue or in providing information when the audience's interest is piqued. Each situation needs to be considered on a case-by-case basis, and practitioners need to be aware that communicating under the guise of a serious health risk can result in heightened and often unnecessary anxiety, especially in environmental and occupational health.[27]

Information needs to be communicated rapidly when there is a need to make control or case subjects in research studies aware of strong evidence that an intervention or treatment is beneficial or harmful.[28] Timing is a consideration when decisions are imminent about public health policies or resource allocations, e.g., during legislative hearings. It can be helpful to communicate information on a topic if it is already receiving a lot of attention among nonscientists because of heightened awareness.[5,29] For example, trends in breast cancer incidence may be of greater interest if they are communicated in conjunction with National Breast Cancer Awareness month.

Public health information can sometimes be communicated in conjunction with unplanned events, such as injury prevention in conjunction with the onset of a natural disaster.[29,30] However, this strategy does not work if the information is not obviously relevant to the event.

Having worked through these planning steps, most communication interventions can be produced and implemented. Recommendations on health communication interventions and campaigns, especially those targeting general public audiences, are well covered in other resources (see, for example, references 3, 4, 5, 23, 29, 31, and 32), and are beyond the scope of this text.

STEP 7: IMPLEMENT THE COMMUNICATION PLAN

After completing the steps 1-6, the next task is to implement the plan by setting in motion the communication activity or activities. Although this step is self-explanatory, it is important to determine if the planned communication activity or activities actually occurred.

STEP 8: EVALUATE THE EFFORT AND ITS IMPACT

The final planning stage involves the evaluation step. Health communication uses formative, process, and outcome (summative) evaluation procedures derived from research in the fields of marketing, psychology, anthropology, public health, and communication. Formative evaluation (pretesting) tasks include researching audience characteristics and testing messages and materials, as described under developing and testing messages (step 4). In addition to the resources listed at the end of the chapter, there are several excellent references available to guide formative evaluation.[31-34] Process and outcome evaluation begin to measure effects higher up the scale suggested by the Hierarchy of Effects Model,[1] although some of this work can be initiated during the formative or pretesting phase. There is an extensive literature on performing process and outcome evaluation for public health programs, much of which is relevant to communication interventions.[35-37]

Process and outcome evaluation attempt to measure whether intended audiences were exposed to messages and to determine if the messages were effective. These evaluations are done most commonly as part of health promotion efforts. Process evaluation assesses the delivery of the communication intervention and measures how well intended audiences were exposed to, attended to, and understood the intended communication messages. Process evaluation is important for attempting to associate communication interventions with potential outcomes, as well as for making mid-course corrections.

An important variable to measure in a process evaluation is "reach," defined as the size of the audience exposed to the message. For a communication intervention to be effective, a large proportion of the target audience (a recent meta-analysis of interventions for the general public suggests about 50%[38]) must be exposed to the message on a frequent basis.[32] Many communication efforts fail simply because the intended audience failed to receive or comprehend the intended message. This can occur in simple situations (e.g., failure of a policy maker to receive a letter) as well as in mass-mediated communication activities (e.g., selecting an inappropriate channel or using a poorly designed message).

In the communication context, outcome evaluation measures changes in knowledge, attitudes, intentions to perform a behavior, or actual health behaviors. Outcomes can be measured in research intervention studies using defined groups (e.g., clinic settings), but there are serious methodological issues when attempting to evaluate the impact of mass communication efforts. For example, it is nearly impossible to have exposed and unexposed treatment and control groups for mass media interventions.[2] Respondents find it very difficult to recall if, when, or where they saw or heard a specific mass media health message. Finally, unplanned events (e.g., news media coverage) can increase exposure or awareness. Because health communication activities are rarely done in isolation from other program interventions, measuring the impact of a selected communication intervention on health outcomes (e.g., morbidity or mortality) is rarely attempted.

OTHER CONSIDERATIONS

To reiterate the broader framework for health communication, it is important to consider other aspects of the problem when planning for communication in public health.

What aspects of the problem or issue are amenable to change through policies, environmental changes, or at the individual level? In what ways could communication contribute to managing the problem or facilitate the desired change? What are others (individuals or organizations) doing? Where are the greatest gaps in communication? What opportunities exist to make a difference? And most importantly, what is reasonable to do given the time available, expertise, and budgetary resources?

EXAMPLES OF APPLYING THE PUBLIC HEALTH COMMUNICATION PLANNING FRAMEWORK

The following five case studies provide examples of applying the public heath communication planning framework described above to "real world" public health situations. The steps are presented as questions that must be answered at each stage of communication planning. Appendix 1 provides a framework guide for readers to use to plan their own communication efforts.

CASE STUDY 1: IMPLEMENTING A NEW SUDDEN INFANT DEATH SYNDROME (SIDS) PREVENTION PROGRAM

A nationwide SIDS public awareness campaign designed to encourage parents to put babies to sleep on their backs is scheduled to occur in two months. The director of a state's maternal and child health (MCH) department would like to use this opportunity to get this message to various audiences such as health care providers and the general public. What steps should be taken to communicate this message?

Step 1: What is the scientific evidence? There is strong evidence from several well-respected research studies demonstrating that infants (under 6 months of age) who sleep on their backs are at decreased risk of death from SIDS.[39,40]

Step 2: Why is communication necessary? The planned communication is proactive. The purpose of the communication is to persuade parents and other child-care givers in the general population to put infants to sleep on their backs.

Step 3: Who is the audience? There are three major target audiences for the communication effort: the general public, health care providers for children, and the news media. The segments of most interest in the general public include families with young infants, pregnant women, and child-care workers. The news media will be encouraged to communicate information to the general public. Health care providers are a secondary audience that can provide messages to infant care givers.

Step 4: What is the message? The fundamental message for health care providers is to encourage patients and family members to always place young infants on their backs to sleep. The message for the news media to be communicated to the general public is: "Back to sleep: reduce your baby's risk of sudden infant death syndrome (SIDS)." Additional information is provided on the number of SIDS deaths per year in the state and that about half of these deaths are preventable.

A preliminary draft of a written brochure (see Step # 5 below) is presented to a selected group of health care providers and 10 parents and family members with young infants (pretesting). Based on feedback from these groups, the language is simplified to the 6th grade reading level, and the brochure is made more visually appealing by bolding key text words and adding clip art to demonstrate proper infant sleeping position.

Step 5: How and where should the message be delivered? Because the primary and secondary target audiences are so concerned about SIDS, a straightforward informational campaign is developed. More elaborate tactics to first gain audience attention are not considered necessary in this case. For health care providers, the Maternal and Child Health department decides to make a series of oral presentations on SIDS prevention at the major child health care institutions in the state and at the annual state pediatrics and family practice conferences. The Department also develops short brochures on how people can prevent SIDS that will be distributed by providers to patients. For the news media, the Department prepares a press release to coincide with the kickoff of the national SIDS prevention campaign, and to develop and provide different story lines to the news media to maintain media interest in the topic. Because of resource constraints, the head of the MCH department decided not to create public service radio or television announcements.

Step 6: When should the message be delivered? Oral presentations to the health care community are to begin as soon as possible. Written brochures and the press release are to be released simultaneously to coincide with the onset of the national campaign to generate maximum media interest.

Step 7: Implement the communication plan. Complete the planned oral presentations to the health care community, provide written brochures to health care providers, and give copies of the press release to news media representatives.

Step 8: Did the audience receive the information and was it effective? For process evaluation the MCH department plans to collect information on the number of health care providers who attend the oral presentations and statewide professional meetings, requests by providers for brochures, and the number of stories about SIDS in state newspapers in the two months following the SIDS prevention campaign. Outcome evaluation will consist of tracking SIDS death rates and near-SIDS hospitalization rates over the next 3 years.

CASE STUDY 2: RISK COMMUNICATION IN A COMMUNITY WITH ASBESTOS IN THE DRINKING WATER

Recent tests of drinking water in a small rural community show abnormally high levels of asbestos. Through news media reports, residents have learned that state health officials have considered advising residents to drink bottled water until the issue is more thoroughly investigated. A public hearing is will be held the next evening to discuss the health issues and the actions that state officials are taking to resolve the problem. The local public health director, who is also a citizen in the community, has been asked to explain the potential health risks and precautionary measures to the county commissioners the next morning, followed by a presentation later that day at the public hearing.

Step 1: What is the scientific evidence? Scientific evidence about the health risks associated with asbestos in drinking water is inconclusive.[41] Nevertheless, the local community is concerned and wants to be assured that their drinking water is safe.

Step 2: Why is communication necessary? This is risk communication and it is reactive (i.e., in response to community requests); the purpose is to inform the audience about this health issue, to address concerns, and to reduce fear among community members.

Step 3: Who is the audience? The audience consists of local elected officials and community residents who use the public water system.

Step 4: What is the message? The message is to describe what is known and unknown about the potential health risks from drinking asbestos-contaminated water, the interim measures to take, and the steps underway to help resolve the issue.

Risk communication is complex and not a common activity for many public health practitioners, so the local health director briefly reviews materials on effective risk communication (chapter 13). Because of the time frame, pretesting is informal and consists of testing the proposed message with a state environmental health official and with the local health official's family members. Based on this feedback, the practitioner minimizes the use of numbers and stresses the actions underway to resolve the issue.

The message is the same for both the elected officials and general public audience. At both meetings, the practitioner must be prepared to acknowledge anxiety and anger, then describe the problem, the magnitude of the potential health risks (e.g., the excess risk of developing cancer is about one in a million among persons who drink two quarts of water per day for 70 years), uncertainty, actions that residents should take, and what is being done to resolve the problem.

Step 5: How and where should the message be delivered? The format for both the elected officials and community members is an oral presentation about the situation.

Step 6: When should the message be delivered? The communication will occur the following day, as the time and day for the presentation have been arranged by others.

Step 7: Implement the communication plan. Make the oral presentations to the meeting of the county commissioners and at the public hearing.

Step 8: Did the audience receive the information and was it effective? Because of lack of resources, no process or outcome evaluation is planned. However, informal discussion with community members provides some feedback.

CASE STUDY 3: ACUTE OUTBREAK OF MEASLES AT A HIGH SCHOOL

Late one afternoon the director of a local health department receives word that two physicians have reported 10 suspected cases of measles among students at the local high school. By the next day, laboratory tests confirm that all of the suspected cases were actually measles.

Step 1: What is the Scientific Evidence? Measles is well-studied, highly contagious infectious disease with potentially serious side effects such as pneumonia and encephalitis.

Vaccinating susceptible individuals (primarily teenagers or young adults), including those who received a single dose many years previously, reduces the risk of disease and continued transmission.[42]

Step 2: Why is communication necessary? This communication is reactive, as it is in response to an acute public health problem. There are several purposes for communicating: to inform individuals about the risk of the problem and precautionary measures to take; to persuade potentially ill patients to visit their health care providers; and to persuade persons potentially at risk for contracting measles to get vaccinated. Additionally, the communication seeks to address fears and concerns among persons in the community.

Step 3: Who is the audience? In this measles outbreak, the audience consists of other students in the school, parents, other members of the general public potentially at risk for contracting measles, school officials, health care providers, health facility administrators, and the news media.

Step 4: What is the message? There are two different messages to communicate to the general public through the news media, school officials, and health care providers: (1) People who have symptoms should notify their health care providers immediately, and (2) persons at risk for measles need to be vaccinated immediately. The two messages for health care providers and health facility administrators are to notify health department officials of suspected cases and to vaccinate patients at risk for measles. Because of the acute nature of the situation, pretesting of messages is only done with professional colleagues.

Step 5: How and where should the message be delivered? The communication channel for reaching the general public is the news media, and this is to be done using a written press release (which includes the name and phone numbers of contact persons at the state and local health departments), and through telephone interviews with the major state newspapers and television stations.

   Although health care providers and health facility administrators can be reached through the news media, a separate one-page written alert is to be mailed, faxed, and e-mailed to them advising them of the outbreak and steps they should undertake. School officials are to be contacted through phone calls, letters, and e-mail about current status and actions they should take. A one-page written document with answers to frequently asked questions about measles is provided so school officials can respond to parents' questions.

Step 6: When should the message be delivered? Once the measles cases are confirmed, the school officials will be notified immediately, followed by the news media and health officials.

Step 7: Implement the communication plan. Provide the press release to the news media and be available for telephone interviews with reporters. The one-page written alert to health care providers is mailed, faxed, and e-mailed to health care providers and health facility administrators. School officials are contacted through phone calls, letters, and e-mail, and provided with the one-page written document with answers to frequently asked questions.

Step 8: Did the audience receive the information and was it effective? Because of the acute nature and need for rapid response process evaluation is not part of planning for outbreaks. Outcome evaluation is straightforward, as it is based on the number of confirmed cases reported after preventive measures have been implemented.

CASE STUDY 4: ENCOURAGING STATE OFFICIALS TO ENACT LEGISLATION TO REDUCE YOUTH ACCESS TO TOBACCO

The governing board of a state voluntary health organization has decided that more needs to be done to reduce youth access to tobacco products. With the support of the governing board, a prominent volunteer in the health organization and the organization's salaried tobacco control director lead an effort to enact state legislation that would ban cigarette vending machines. Such an effort will be a difficult struggle against the tobacco and vending machine industry lobbies.

Step 1: What is the scientific evidence? There is a large body of evidence demonstrating that most persons who become regular smokers begin smoking prior to age 18.[43] National, state, and local surveys indicate that most youth have little difficulty purchasing cigarettes from vending machines, and that vending machines can be used by youth to obtain cigarettes, although other sources are more popular.[43]

Step 2: Why is communication necessary? The purpose of this proactive health communication is to persuade elected officials (state legislators) to enact legislation to effect an environmental change that will make it more difficult for adolescents to obtain cigarettes.

Step 3: Who is the audience? Although the entire legislature is the intended audience, efforts are first directed to two legislators known to be sympathetic to tobacco control activities. Secondary audiences include the state public health association and the state medical society (to garner additional support), and the news media to generate interest and support for the legislation among other constituencies and the general public.

Step 4: What is the message? Pretesting messages is vitally important in legislative advocacy, so the tobacco control director shares the draft legislation with the organization's lobbyist and other persons knowledgeable about legislative language and the approaches needed to help increase the likelihood of passage. The final message consists of data on the percent of underage smokers in the state who have used a cigarette vending machine and that banning cigarette vending machines will reduce access to these products.

Step 5: How and where should the message be delivered? Obtaining access and gaining interest of legislators is important but difficult, and the legislative process complex, so the tobacco control director works with the voluntary health organization's lobbyist. They develop a one-page written summary that highlights key facts about youth and cigarette vending machines in the state (e.g., the percent of youth in the state who have used a cigarette vending machine, and the expected impact of the proposed law in reducing sales to youth).

The tobacco control director prepares a five to 10 minute oral presentation for a committee hearing that includes the points mentioned above. For the presentation, he creates a short videotape that shows very young children purchasing cigarettes from vending machines, and he has an underage smoker prepare testimony on the ease and importance of vending machines for obtaining cigarettes for himself and his friends. The news media (major state newspaper and television reporters) will be notified prior to the hearing and provided copies of the videotape and the written testimony.

Step 6: When should the message be delivered? Successful legislative advocacy begins before the legislative session, so the tobacco control director arranges meetings with aides to key legislators and representatives of potential supporting organizations. Because of the tight time lines for most state legislatures, further meetings will be arranged with key legislators and organization representatives very early in the legislative session to keep the issue at the forefront.

Step 7: Implement the communication plan. The tobacco control director completes his short oral presentation, shows the videotape of the young children successfully purchasing cigarettes from vending machines, and has the young smoker provide his testimony. He also provides the one-page written summary to the committee and to news media representatives.

Step 8: Did the audience receive the information and was it effective? Only a simple process evaluation is planned that will consist of tracking the number of meetings with legislators and the number of news stories about cigarette vending machines. The outcome evaluation consists of seeing if the legislation passes, if the law is enforced, and if youth access to tobacco through vending machines is reduced over the next two years (i.e., through surveys).

CASE STUDY 5: ADVOCATING FOR RESOURCES WITHIN A PRIVATE HEALTH ORGANIZATION

After reviewing a series of reports and articles on the leading causes of childhood mortality and morbidity, an employee of a health maintenance organization (HMO) becomes convinced that the organization needs to focus more efforts on childhood injury prevention; no resources are currently being devoted to this topic.

Step 1: What is the scientific evidence? There is a wealth of evidence demonstrating that injuries are the predominant health problem for children in the United States.[44,45]

Step 2: Why is communication necessary? The purpose of this communication is to acquire resources to begin an injury prevention program. The communication is proactive and the employee must persuade the chief administrator to fund the program.

Step 3: Who is the audience? The chief administrator of the HMO.

Step 4: What is the message? The message is that an injury prevention program can save lives, reduce the risk of hospitalization, and result in reduced use of health care resources. The employee pretests her message by asking several colleagues to review her proposal and listen to her presentation. She does this to make sure her proposal covers the essential items and is likely to get the administrator's attention. She also asks her colleagues to provide feedback as to the form of presentation preferred by the administrator.

The information to be presented briefly covers the extent of the childhood injury problem, data on injury hospitalizations, estimated costs to the HMO, the effectiveness of interventions (e.g., bicycle helmets and child motor vehicle restraints), the budget for the new program, and the anticipated cost savings to the HMO based on the program.

Step 5: How and where should the message be delivered? The information is condensed into a one-page written summary and includes a bulleted list to highlight key points. Because the employee only has 10 minutes with the administrator, she prepares a 5 minute oral presentation that will stress the key aspects of her proposal and she allows 5 minutes for questions. The oral presentation includes a simple bar chart and pie chart that visually highlight the injury burden and cost implications to the HMO.

Step 6: When should the message be delivered? The proposal for a new program should be presented to the administrator early in the budget preparation process. The presentation should be postponed if other pressing issues distract the administrator.

Step 7: Implement the communication plan. The HMO employee does the oral presentation for the HMO administrator and provides him with the one-page bulleted summary.

Step 8: Did the audience receive the information and was it effective? Process evaluation is not relevant. Outcome evaluation is not necessary as the success of the proposal will be evident within a short time.

SUMMARY

Despite the multiple opportunities and situations, communication planning consists of eight steps: assessing the science, defining the purpose (why), identifying and understanding the audience(s) (who), developing and testing message concepts (what), choosing media and channels for message delivery (how and where), determining the best timing for delivering the message (when), implementing the communication plan, and evaluating the effort and impact (effectiveness).

The purpose behind the communication is to inform or persuade audiences that consist of either individuals or policy makers. Audience considerations include demographics and other personal characteristics; level of involvement and readiness to change; and primary, secondary, and tertiary audiences. Message development will vary, depending on the purpose and audience, but messages need to be simple and readily understood. Pretesting of message content and delivery with the intended audience can greatly enhance communication efforts.

Media and communication channels include interpersonal contact, written materials and audiovisuals, mass media, and electronic media. The timing of communication varies greatly depending on circumstances. Process evaluation is used to measure whether the information was disseminated as planned and if it was received, understood, and remembered by the intended audience. Outcome evaluation attempts to measure the decision-making or health behavior change in response to communication interventions.

Planning is critical for public health communication. By making a serious effort to understand audiences, messages that are likely to resonate, the channels likely to reach them, and evaluating effectiveness, practitioners are much more likely to effectively communicate messages and achieve improvements in population health.

CHAPTER 2 ENDNOTES

1. McGuire WJ. Theoretical foundations of campaigns. In: Rice RE, Atkin CK, editors. *Public Communication Campaigns*. 2nd ed. Beverly Hills, CA: Sage Publications; 1989: 43-65.

2. Freimuth VS, Cole G, Kirby S. Issues in evaluating mass mediated health communication campaigns. In: Rootman I, Goodstadt M, Hyndman B, McQueen DV, Potvin L, Springett J, et al. eds. *Evaluation in Health Promotion: Principles and Perspectives*. Geneva: WHO Regional Publications, European Series, No. 92, 2001.

3. Centers for Disease Control and Prevention. *CDCynergy 2001: Your Guide to Effective Health Communication*. Atlanta, GA: CDC Office of Communication; 2001.

4. USDHHS, National Cancer Institute. *Making health communication programs work: A planner's guide*. NIH Publication No. 92-1493; 1992. Available at: http://oc.nci.nih.gov/services/hcpw/home.htm.

5. Siegel M, Doner L. *Marketing Public Health. Strategies to Promote Social Change*. Gaithersburg, MD: Aspen; 1998.

6. Research America. Porter/Novelli "HealthStyles" survey, 1998 and1999.

7. Institute of Medicine and National Research Council. *Exposure of the American people to Iodine-131 from Nevada nuclear-bomb tests. Review of the National Cancer Institute Report and public health implications*. Washington, DC: *National Academy Press*; 1999.

8. Russell C. Hype, hysteria, and women's health risks: the role of the media. *Women's Health Issues* 1993;3(4):191-197.

9. Andreasen A, ed. *Ethics in social marketing*. Washington, DC: Georgetown University Press; 2001.

10. Society for Public Health Education (SOPHE). Code of Ethics for the Health Education Profession. *Health Educ Behav.* 2002; 29:11.

11. Terris, M. The Society of Epidemiologic Research (SER) and the future of epidemiology. *Am J Epidemiol* 1992;136:909-915.

12. Witte K. The manipulative nature of health communication research. *Am Behav Scientist* 1994;38:285-293.

13. Andreasen AR. *Marketing Social Change: Changing Behavior to Promote Health, Social Development and the Environment.* San Francisco, CA: Jossey-Bass; 1995.

14. Weinstein A. *Market Segmentation.* Chicago, IL: Probus; 1994.

15. Maibach EW, Maxfield A, Ladin K, Slater M. Translating health psychology into effective health communication: the American healthstyles audience segmentation project. *J Health Psychol* 1996;1:261-277.

16. Slater MD. Choosing audience segmentation strategies and methods for health communication. In: Maibach EW and Parrott RL, eds, *Designing Health Messages*. Newbury Park , CA: Sage; 1995: 186-198.

17. Bandura A. *Social Learning Theory.* Englewood Cliffs, NJ: Prentice Hall; 1977.

18. Lyon-Daniels K, Prue C. "Ready, Not Ready": Developing a targeted campaign to increase pre-natal folic acid consumption. Society for Public Health Education Annual Meeting. June 1999; Washington, DC.

19. Prochaska JO, DiClemente CC, Norcross JC. In search of how people change: Applications to addictive behaviors. *Am Psychol* 1992; 47:1102-1114.

20. Maibach EW, Cotton D. Moving People to Behavior Change: A Staged Social Cognitive Approach to Message Design. In: Maibach EW, Parrott RL, eds, *Designing Health Messages*. Newbury Park, CA: Sage; 1995: 41-64.

21. Brislin RW, Yoshida T. *Improving Intercultural Interactions: Modules for Cross-Cultural Training Programs.* Thousand Oaks, CA: Sage; 1994.

22. Huff RM, Kline MV. *Promoting Health in Multicultural Populations. A Handbook for Practitioners.* Thousand Oaks, CA: Sage;1999.

23. Kreuter MW, Lezin NA, Kreuter MW, Green LW. *Community Health Promotion. Ideas that Work. A field-book for practitioners.* Sudbury, MA: Jones and Bartlett; 1998.

24. Kreuter MW, Farrell D, Olevitch L, Brennan L. *Tailoring Health Messages: Customizing Communication Using Computer Technology.* Mahwah, NJ: Lawrence Erlbaum Associates; 1999.

25. Blalock SJ, DeVellis BM, Patterson CC, Campbell MK, Orenstein DR, Dooley MA. Effects of an osteoporosis prevention program incorporating tailored educational materials. *Am J Health Promot.* 2002; 16:146-56.

26. Public Health Emergency Preparedness and Response. Available at: http://www.bt.cdc.gov.
27. Kulldorff M, Feuer EJ, Miller BA, Freedman LS. Breast Cancer clusters in the northeast United States: a geographic analysis. *Am J Epidemiol* 1997;146:161-170.
28. Coughlin JF Beacahmp TL. *Ethics and Epidemiology.* New York: Oxford; 1996.
29. Wallack L, Dorfman L, Jernigan D, Themba M. *Media Advocacy and Public Health.* Newbury Park, CA: Sage; 1993.
30. Shattuck T. Lecture-medicine and the media. *N Eng J Med* 1998;339:161-170.
31. USAID. *A Toolbox for Building Health Communication Capacity.* Washington, DC: Academy for Educational Development, BASICS Project; 1996.
32. Hornik R. Public health communication: making sense of contradictory evidence. In: Hornik R, ed. *Public Health Communication: Evidence for Behavior Change.* Mahwah, NJ: Erlbaum; 2002.
33. Krueger RA. *Focus Groups: A Practical guide for Applied Research. 2nd ed.* Upper Saddle River, NJ: Prentice-Hall; 1994.
34. Morse JM, Field PA. *Qualitative Research Methods for Health Professionals. 2nd ed.* Thousand Oaks, CA: Sage; 1995.
35. Thompson NJ, McClintock HO. *Demonstrating your program's worth. A primer on evaluation for programs to prevent unintentional injury.* Atlanta: Centers for Disease Control and Prevention, NCIPC;1998.
36. Patton MQ. *Utilization-Focused Evaluation: The New Century Text, 3rd ed.* Thousand Oaks ,CA: Sage; 1997.
37. Herman JL, Morris LL, Fitz-Gibbon CT. *Evaluator's Handbook.* Newbury Park, CA: Sage; 1987.
38. Snyder LB. How effective are mediated campaigns? In Rice R, & Atkin C, eds: *Public Information Campaigns. 3rd ed.* Thousand Oaks, CA: Sage; 2000.
39. Henderson-Smart DJ, Ponsonby AI, Murphy E. Reducing the risk of SIDS: a scientific review of the literature. *J Paediatr Child Health* 1998;34:213-219.
40. American Academy of Pediatrics and Selected Agencies of the Federal Government. Infant sleep position and sudden infant death syndrome (SIDS) in the United States [joint commentary]. *Pediatrics* 1994;93:820.
41. Gamble JF Asbestos and cancer: a weight-of-the-evidence review. *Environ Health Perspect* 1994;102:1038-1050.
42. Atkinson WL, Pickering LK, Schwartz B, Weniger BG, Iskander JK, Watson JC. General Recommendations on Immunization: Recommendations of the Advisory Committee on Immunization Practices (ACIP) and the American Academy of Family Physicians (AAFP). *MMWR Recomm Rep.* 2002;51(RR02):1-36.
43. U.S. Department of Health and Human Services. *Preventing Tobacco Use Among Young People: A Report of the Surgeon General.* Atlanta, GA: U.S. Department of Health and Human Services, Public Health Service, Centers for Disease Control and Prevention, National Center for Chronic Disease Prevention and Health Promotion, Office on Smoking and Health; 1994.
44. Institute of Medicine. *Injury in America.* Washington, DC: National Academy Press; 1985.
45. CDC. *Health, United States 2001, With Urban and Rural Chartbook.* Hyattsville, MD: CDC, National Center for Health Statistics; 2001.

SUGGESTED READINGS AND RESOURCES

Centers for Disease Control and Prevention. *CDCynergy 2001: Your Guide to Effective Health Communication.* Atlanta: CDC Office of Communication; 2001.

Huff RM, Kline MV, Eds. *Promoting Health in Multicultural Populations. A Handbook for Practitioners.* Thousand Oaks, CA: Sage; 1999.

Kreuter M, Lezin NA, Kreuter MW, Green LW. *Community Health Promotion Ideas that Work. A Field-Book for Practitioners.* Sudbury, MA: Jones and Bartlett;1998.

Siegel M, Doner L. *Marketing Public Health: Strategies to Promote Social Change.* Gaithersburg, MD: Aspen; 1998.

USDHHS, National Cancer Institute, 1992. *Making Health Communication Programs Work: A Planners Guide.* NIH Publication No. 92-1493. Available at: http://oc.nci.nih.gov/services/hcpw/home.htm.

Windsor R, Baranowski T, Clark N, Cutte G. *Evaluation of Health Promotion, Health Education and Disease Prevention Programs. 2nd ed.* Mountain View, CA: Mayfield; 1994.

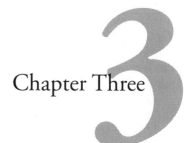

Chapter Three

TRANSLATING PUBLIC HEALTH DATA

David E. Nelson, M.D., M.P.H.

I t was Hippocrates who said "There are in fact two things: science and opinion. One begets knowledge, the latter ignorance."[1] One of the biggest challenges in public health communication is locating timely and trustworthy scientific information and effectively translating the numbers, scientific reasoning, and mathematical concepts to non-scientific audiences.

BACKGROUND

Public health information that is communicated to nonscientists fundamentally depends on high quality science, which involves the collection, analysis, and interpretation of data. Scientists understand hypothesis testing, mathematics, uncertainty, the iterative nature of the scientific approach, and the caveats of public health surveillance data sets and research studies. Communication with scientific audiences about public health data generally involves describing methodology, presenting substantial amounts of data, and discussing uncertainty and limitations.

In contrast, most nonscientific audiences are not well-versed in mathematics or science;[2] they often rely on anecdotes, recommendations from friends or relatives, or personal experience when making decisions about their health.[3] Communicating data to nonscientists differs markedly from that of communicating with scientists; nonscientists want the bottom line about what the findings show, what they mean, and as a result, what should be done.

LOCATING PUBLIC HEALTH DATA AND OTHER SCIENTIFIC INFORMATION

Thanks to the ever-expanding science base and improvements in technology (e.g., the Internet), data and other forms of information are now easily available, although locating high-quality, reliable information remains a challenge.

There are five major sources for locating written scientific information: books, scientific journals, annual or periodic reports, CD-ROMs, and the Internet. Books and journals remain a fundamental source for information, especially research findings. Because of the diversity of topics and the large number of publications, a listing of suggested public health publications is beyond the scope of this book (readers are referred to reference 4 for a further discussion of suggested epidemiology books and journals).

The most common databases for searching the public health literature are MEDLINE, PsychINFO, Sociological Abstracts, Embase, Current Contents (Clinical Medicine, Life Sciences, or Social and Behavioral Sciences), HealthSTAR, Popline, Institute for Scientific Information (ISI) Web of Science, Combined Health Information Database (CHID), Toxline, and Cancerlit. Access to one or more of these databases can usually be obtained through public or private libraries, government agencies, or universities, and several can be searched at no charge through the National Library of Medicine or other federal Web sites[5] (Table 3.1). There are document retrieval services that help locate and retrieve articles, documents, and books,[6, 7] and increasingly, complete journal articles can be obtained from Web sites.

TABLE 3.1—SELECTED INTERNET WEB SITE ADDRESSES FOR SEARCHING THE PUBLIC HEALTH LITERATURE

Name of Data Base	Internet Web Site
PubMed	http://www.ncbi.nlm.nih.gov/PubMed
MedlinePlus	http://www.nlm.nih.gov/medlineplus
Cancerlit	http://www.cancer.gov/search/cancer_literature/
Combined Health Information Database (CHID)	http://chid.nih.gov/

Table 3.2 contains a selected list of annual and periodic publications with public health surveillance data and summaries of research findings. *Health, United States* and the *Statistical Abstract of the United States*, both of which are published annually, are especially valuable resources.[8,9] Many state and local health departments also routinely publish public health data and other information in annual reports and newsletters. CD-ROMS, because of their storage capacity, are often used to make available public health data and other information gathered from databases, reports, etc.; a number of these CD-ROMS are available from the CDC,[10-12] the Agency for Healthcare Research and Quality (AHRQ),[13] and the U.S. Census Bureau.[14] (Information for obtaining CD-ROMs from these and other agencies can be obtained from Web site addresses listed in Appendix 2.)

The Internet has fostered substantial advances in locating public health data in recent years. Materials that were once difficult to obtain (the "gray" or "fugitive" literature) are increasingly available on Web sites. Large documents and reports can now be easily and rapidly downloaded onto personal computers, and in some instances, Internet Web sites have replaced CD-ROMS as a way to access databases. For example, it is possible to directly query certain databases through Web sites from the U.S. Census Bureau and National Center for Health Statistics to conduct descriptive data analyses.[11,14]

There are tens of thousands of health-related Web sites.[15,16] Unfortunately, the quality of scientific information available from Internet sites is highly variable,[16] and Web site addresses frequently change, making locating information difficult. Appendix 2 contains a

TABLE 3.2—SELECTED ROUTINE AND PERIODIC PUBLICATIONS WITH PUBLIC HEALTH DATA

Publication	Source	Web Site Address for Obtaining Publications
Published several times per year		
Morbidity and Mortality Weekly Report (MMWR) and Surveillance Summaries	Centers for Disease Control and Prevention (CDC)	http://www.cdc.gov/mmwr
National Vital Statistics Report (NVSR)	CDC's National Center for Health Statistics (NCHS)	http://www.cdc.gov/nchs/products/pubs/pubd/nvsr/nvsr.htm
Advance Data from Vital and Health Statistics	NCHS	http://www.cdc.gov/nchs/products/pubs/pubd/ad/ad.htm
State and local health department newsletters	State and local health departments†	Various; see Appendix 2 for list of state health department web sites
Health, United States	NCHS	http://www.cdc.gov/nchs/hus.htm
Annual state health data reports	State health departments†	Various; see Appendix 2 for list of state health department web sites
Statistical Abstract of the United States	U.S. Bureau of the Census	http://www.census.gov/statab/www
State and Metropolitan Area Data Book	U.S. Bureau of the Census	http://www.census.gov/statab/www/smadb.html
State Health Profiles	CDC	Available via email: shprofiles@cdc.gov
Current Population Reports: Health Insurance	U.S. Bureau of the Census	http://www.census.gov/hhes/www/hlthins.html
National Household Survey on Drug Abuse: Population Estimates and Main Findings, and other reports on alcohol, tobacco, and illegal drug use	Substance Abuse and Mental Health Services Administration (SAMHSA)	http://www.drugabusestatistics.samhsa.gov
World Health Report and other publications	World Health Organization (WHO)	http://www3.who.int/whosis/menu.cfm
Behavioral Risk Factor Surveillance System (BRFSS) Summary Prevalence Report	CDC	http://www.cdc.gov/nccdphp/brfss
Apparent Per Capita Alcohol Consumption: National, State, and Regional Trends	National Institutes of Health (NIH), National Institute on Alcohol Abuse and Alcoholism (NIAAA)	http://www.niaaa.nih.gov/publications/surveillance.htm

Publication	Source	Web Site Address for Obtaining Publications
Health Resources and Services Administration (HRSA) State Profiles	HRSA	http://www.hrsa.gov/data.htm
Cancer Facts and Figures	American Cancer Society	http://www.cancer.org/eprise/main/docroot/stt/stt_0
Injury Facts	National Safety Council	http://www.nsc.org/lrs/statstop.htm
Heart and Stroke Statistical Update	American Heart Association	http://www.americanheart.org/statistics
Intermittent Publications		
Surgeon General Reports on Tobacco	U.S. Department of Health and Human Services (USDHHS)	http://www.cdc.gov/tobacco
Reports to Congress on Alcohol and Health	USDHHS, NIH, NIAAA	http://www.niaaa.nih.gov/publications/publications.htm
Consensus Development Statements	NIH	http://odp.od.nih.gov/consensus/cons/cons.htm
Data from the National Health Interview Survey ("Rainbow" Series 10)	NCHS	http://www.cdc.gov/nchs/products/pubs/pubd/series/sr10/ser10.htm
Data on Health Resources Utilization ("Rainbow" Series 13)	NCHS	http://www.cdc.gov/nchs/products/pubs/pubd/series/sr13/ser13.htm
Data on Natality, Marriage, and Divorce ("Rainbow" Series 21)	NCHS	http://www.cdc.gov/nchs/products/pubs/pubd/series/sr21/ser21.htm
SEER Cancer Statistics Review	NIH, National Cancer Institute	http://seer.cancer.gov
National Health Objectives (Healthy People 2010)	USDHHS	http://www.health.gov/healthypeople
U.S. Preventive Services Task Force Guide to Clinical Preventive Services	USDHHS, Office of Disease Prevention and Health Promotion	http://www.ahrq.gov/clinic/prevnew.htm

selected list of Web sites (primarily from federal agencies) that are reliable sources for locating data and other information useful for public health practice. Appendix 2 is by no means comprehensive, but these Web sites are likely to be consistently maintained and updated. Although many of the sites in Appendix 2 have such information, state health departments are likely to be better sources for state or local data; Appendix 3 contains Web site addresses for state health departments. Note, however, that state health department Web site addresses often change more frequently than those for federal agencies or from private health organizations, and Internet directories and search engines may be necessary to locate current Web site addresses.

TRANSLATING PUBLIC HEALTH DATA: GENERAL CONSIDERATIONS

The amount and complexity of information to communicate to nonscientific audiences will vary widely and depend upon the purpose of the communication and the audience. However, several general considerations are applicable for most situations.

ASSESS THE QUALITY OF THE SCIENCE

As introduced in the previous chapter, appropriately assessing the science is the first step when considering communicating public data and other information to nonscientists.[17,18] Examples of assessing the science include examining the study design, quality of data collection, representativeness of populations, sensitivity and specificity of tests, statistical analyses, and interpretation of findings. For example, there can be a temptation to overinterpret or overgeneralize scientific findings,[19-21] especially with the strong bias for reporting positive results; one study or report is rarely the definitive work.

The credibility of the presenter and the circumstances under which the findings are introduced to audiences are additional considerations. The credibility of those presenting scientific findings should be carefully examined for potential conflicts of interest or ulterior motives.[21,22] Research sponsored by tobacco companies, pharmaceutical corporations, and advocacy groups are just a few examples where credibility can be a problem. Be wary of findings that are solely based on presentations at conferences, in organizational reports, or on Web sites (excluding peer-reviewed electronic journals published solely on-line). Peer review results in delays in publication, but provides some level of assurance that other scientists consider the findings worthy of publication. Though imperfect, it is the closest approach to a "gold standard" for scientific evidence. The timing of when information is released needs to be scrutinized, as some individuals and organizations widely publicize data that coincides with policy deliberations or legislative votes.

Tables 3.3 and 3.4 provide an overview of questions to ask and factors to consider when assessing the quality of the science.[19,20,23]

TABLE 3.3—QUESTIONS TO ASK ABOUT DATA ANALYSES AND DATA QUALITY

Is it a problem?
How do they know?
If it's a problem, how great or small is it, and under what circumstances?
Are these data preliminary?
What are the limitations of these data?
What's missing?
Does the statistical evidence back the conclusions?
What is the degree of certainty or uncertainty?
What are the alternative explanations?
Does a correlation suggest a causal association?
Could the relationship described be explained by other factors?
Have there been any (or any other) studies or experiments?
Have results been consistent from study to study?
Have the findings resulted in a consensus among others in the field?
Should judgment be withheld until there is more evidence?

Adapted from Reference 19

TABLE 3.4—CONSIDERATIONS FOR EVALUATING THE QUALITY OF PUBLIC HEALTH RESEARCH FINDINGS	
Less Certain	More Certain
One of a few observations	Many observations
Anecdote or case reports	Scientific study
Not published	Published in peer-reviewed journal
Not previously reported	Reproduces findings from other studies
Nonhuman subjects	Human subjects
Results not related to hypotheses	Results related to tested hypotheses
No limitations mentioned	Limitations mentioned
Not compared to previous results	Relationship to previous studies discussed

Adapted from reference 23

A full understanding of how to assess the quality of the science behind public health requires extensive training in statistics and other graduate-level courses. It has been the subject of hundreds of books and articles and is beyond the scope of this book. The text *Studying a Study and Testing a Test* (reference 18) is an excellent introduction to this topic.

PRESENT DATA ETHICALLY

Because public health practitioners are often perceived as experts by nonscientists, practitioners have an important responsibility to act ethically when communicating quantitative information to nonscientific audiences.[24]

Improper presentations of data are a daily occurrence in the business and political world,[20-22] such as when skewed graphs of corporate earnings are used to pacify stockholders or when exaggerations (worst-case scenarios) of projected cost are used to oppose legislative bills. Unfortunately, public health professionals have been guilty of similar errors.[20] Public health data must be communicated honestly, regardless of the "justness" of the issue, as most people are aware that data can be manipulated and do not blindly trust numbers.[19,22,25] Often data are conflicting or inconclusive; when this happens, it is best to admit it and say, "I don't know." Although nonscientific audiences usually want definitive answers or solutions, in public health such answers can be elusive.

Overinterpretation and overgeneralization are especially common ethical problems. Small increases or decreases in incidence or prevalence of health conditions occur all too commonly and can be manipulated for specific purposes.[20,22] For example, a change in prevalence from 1% to 2% can be described as a two-fold (or 100%) increase. Although mathematically correct, such a description can be misleading, as the absolute increase is only 1 percentage point, and because most nonscientific audiences are unaware of the distinction between absolute and relative percent difference.[19,20] Misleading visual displays are another common form of misusing data to demonstrate desired results[20,26] (chapter 11).

BE SELECTIVE IN THE USE OF DATA

To prevent confusion, it is important to be highly selective and present only the key data to nonscientists.[25,27-29] In contrast to scientific audiences, who are usually familiar with numbers and often expect them to be used to justify statements, nonscientists rarely want to be presented much data. The one exception to this recommendation is presenting cost data to elected officials and administrators, when communicating more detailed information about data (or being prepared to do so) is often desirable.

Although scientific data provide the objective basis for public health action, it is important to recall that data are only one of many factors individuals use to process information and make decisions. Other considerations include personal experience, financial incentives, or anecdotes.[3,30,31]

CONSIDER DATA THAT WILL BE OF INTEREST TO THE AUDIENCE

Although the specifics will vary by audience, it is necessary to consider magnitude, context, meaning, and action when communicating public health data. Answering several questions can help practitioners decide what data are likely to be of greatest interest to nonscientific audiences (Table 3.5).[19,28,29,31]

The first consideration is magnitude. How big a problem is this? How does the magnitude and importance of this problem compare with other problems affecting the audience? Consider the number of people involved or affected (or potentially affected), the types of individuals (e.g., children, special populations), the extent of the risk or benefit (e.g., to mortality, morbidity, quality of life, regular activities), and the costs involved in addressing or failing to address the problem. Administrators and elected officials are especially likely to focus on cost-related issues.

In what context is this problem occurring? How do these data compare with data elsewhere (locally, statewide, nationally, internationally)? How do these data compare with other groups of people; for example, are there demographic disparities such as differences

TABLE 3.5—CONSIDERATIONS FOR DECIDING WHAT DATA TO PRESENT TO NONSCIENTIFIC AUDIENCES	
Magnitude	How big a problem is this? How does the size and importance of this problem compare with other problems affecting the audience?
Context	How do these data compare with data elsewhere (e.g., locally, statewide, nationally, internationally)? How do these data compare with other groups of people—for example, are there sociodemographic disparities, such as differences by age, sex, or race/ethnicity? Is the health problem getting better, worse, or staying the same over time—that is, is there a trend?
Meaning	Is the problem preventable? Is the audience, or are their friends or family, personally at risk for experiencing a health problem? Will the audience be held accountable for addressing the problem?
Action	As a result of these findings, what needs to be done? Will further information be forthcoming, how will the audience get it, and when will it be available?

Adapted from References 2, 19, 20, 28, 29, and 31

by age, sex, or race/ethnicity? For surveillance data, what are the trends? Is the health problem getting better, worse, or staying the same over time?[19,22] Reporting that there were 167 cases of measles in the first half of 1993 was more meaningful when it also communicated that this was a 99% decrease from the more than 13,000 cases reported in the first half of 1990.[32]

Consider what these data mean for the specific audience.[20,31] Is the audience, or are their friends or families, personally at risk for experiencing this particular health problem or are they being held accountable for addressing the problem? Is this problem preventable?

Given these data, what actions need to be taken? This could include actions taken by the persons in the audience themselves, by other individuals, government agencies, private businesses, administrators, or elected officials. The actions could range from doing nothing, to monitoring the situation, to using specific preventive measures, to recommending increases in personnel or funding, to encouraging enactment or rescission of a specific policy. Finally, will further information be forthcoming, and how and when will it be provided?

SIMPLIFY DATA AND EXPLAIN UNFAMILIAR TERMS AND CONCEPTS

Many nonscientific audiences have low mathematical literacy,[2] including highly-educated persons.[33,34] Even nonscientists who are well-versed in math rarely have the time to closely examine numbers. Terms and concepts commonly used in public health, such as incidence, prevalence, rates, ratios, relative risk, attributable risk, and risk assessment, are unfamiliar to most nonscientists and need to be simplified for many audiences.[35] Even percentages are not well understood by many members of the general public.[2,33,36]

Whenever possible, public health data terms and concepts need to be explained in ways that are familiar to the audience. When presenting information about relative risk, it is better to state that "smoking cigarettes doubles the risk of dying from a heart attack" rather than presenting a relative risk of 2.0.[37,38] Similarly, with percentages, a phrase such as "1 out of every 4 adults does not wear a safety belt" is preferable to stating that 25% of adults do not wear safety belts.[36,37]

Communicating rates to nonscientific audiences, especially the general public and the news media, can be challenging. Incidence, prevalence, mortality, and birth rates are common public health terms but are not easily translated to low-numeracy audiences. One approach is to describe rates as how many people currently have a health condition out of a population of 100,000.[36] An even better approach is to try and convert rates into actual numbers of people, as in stating that in a certain state [or city] there were "x" persons who became sick with condition "y" during the previous year. If the rates are fairly high, the numbers of persons can be compared to the total population of a city or region to help provide context (i.e., "The number of alcohol-impaired drivers on the road this weekend was larger than the total population of Smithville, the state's 6th largest city."). This comparison is an example of a numeric analogy, which is discussed further in the next section.

There are times, however, when more detailed explanations about data and epidemiologic concepts are needed. This is especially true when explaining risk factors or when doing risk communication[39] (chapter 13). At such times, mathematical and scientific terms and concepts unfamiliar to the audience must be introduced carefully and thoroughly explained before presenting data.[28,29] This level of detail is needed regardless of the form or channel of communication. For example, the concept of risk factors, lifetime risk, and confidence intervals would need to be clearly explained before communicating a message about the lifetime risk of breast cancer, such as "If there were 100 women who shared these same risk factors, 11 of them would have a 95% chance of being diagnosed with breast cancer sometime in their life."

CREATE RELEVANT NUMERIC ANALOGIES

Numeric analogies, sometimes referred to as "creative epidemiology" or "social math," can be used to translate health data into terms that are comprehensible, meaningful, and personalized to the intended audience.[31,38,40] Numeric analogies date back at least to the 19th century (e.g., "The world's production of beer for 1894 was nearly 52 billion gallons. Beer kegs sufficient to hold this quality would belt the earth seven times at the equator."[31,41]). Analogies are often used by skilled science writers and speakers.[28,29,31] One of the most commonly cited numeric analogy examples in public health is that the number of deaths from cigarette smoking in the United States is equivalent to the number of deaths that would occur if 2 jumbo jets crashed every day with no survivors.[31,37,38]

Numeric analogies can be used for many public health issues, and they can be used for both reactive and proactive communication. Table 3.6 contains specific examples that illustrate numeric analogies. Developing the analogies can be challenging, but there are several principles to help guide their creation.[40]

First, use numbers based on short time periods. It is more effective to describe the number of deaths or persons diagnosed within an hour or a day than to present the number occurring over one or more years. Second, compare numbers to a specific place familiar to the audience, such as a university, hospital, or city. Third, compare numbers to something that the audience can readily grasp, as in the number of firearms dealers relative to the number of McDonald's restaurants. Fourth, use irony: for example, compare average hourly wages for child-care workers with wages for prison guards. Fifth, try to personalize numbers for the audience, such as stating that in this community, 6 out of 10 people will eventually die from cardiovascular disease or cancer.

Numeric analogies can provide an easy hook for remembering a key message point, but they must be based on actual data. To be most effective, numeric analogies should be localized and personalized to the audience because meaning and impact may not transfer readily from one audience to the next (Box 3.1).[31,42]

BOX 3.1

An employee working for the state substance abuse prevention program would like to gain the interest and support of school superintendents for new anti-tobacco and anti-alcohol education curricula. He reviews recent estimates from the state's Youth Risk Behavior Survey (YRBS).[10] YRBS data indicate that current smoking prevalence among high school students in the state increased from 25% to 35% during the 1990s, and that 38% of students consumed 5 or more alcoholic beverages on one or more occasions during the past 30 days. To get the attention of the superintendents and to personalize the magnitude of these problems, he prepares a short oral presentation and 1 page handout with data. Based on the state's YRBS data, he provides school district-specific estimates of the number of students who will begin smoking each year and the number of students who will engage in binge drinking each month.

TABLE 3.6—EXAMPLES OF NUMERIC ANALOGIES

Tobacco	1,000 people quit smoking every day—by dying. That is the equivalent of 2 fully loaded jumbo jets crashing every day with no survivors. Each year, more than 1 million children begin smoking; this is the equivalent of 33,000 classrooms per year or 90 classrooms every day.
Alcohol	College students consume enough alcohol to fill 3,500 Olympic-size swimming pools, or about 1 swimming pool on every campus in the United States. The alcohol industry spends approximately $225,000 every hour of every day to advertise and promote alcohol consumption. Rhode Island, with 3 times the population of South Central Los Angeles, has 220 liquor stores. By comparison, South Central Los Angeles has 728 liquor stores.
Nutrition	Medium-sized buttered popcorn at the theater contains more artery-clogging fat than a bacon and eggs breakfast, a Big Mac and fries for lunch, and a steak dinner with all the trimmings....combined.
Firearms	There are 10 times as many gun dealers in California as there are McDonald's restaurants.
Child health	Child health care workers make less than $10 per hour, whereas prison guards are paid more than $18 per hour.
Health care reform	Only 3% of Canadians would prefer a U.S. private health insurance model to the Single Payer model. Put in perspective, 16% of Canadians believe that Elvis Presley is still alive.
Infectious Diseases	Every weekend, more than 16,000 teenagers will be infected with a sexually transmitted disease.

Sources: References 31, 36, 40

TRANSLATING PUBLIC HEALTH DATA: RECOMMENDED FORMATS

Of the many ways to describe and present public health data, only a few are likely to be effective with nonscientific audiences. The first consideration is whether data should be presented at all. Again, given the problems that many general public audiences have with numbers, presenting no data may be the best choice for the general public, and practitioners may be best served by communicating only the nature of the health problem and the recommended course of action.

If data are to be communicated, the best approach is often to simply present the numbers of persons affected by the public health problem. The numbers can be actual counts (e.g., the number of deaths associated with a hurricane), estimates based on population-based surveys (e.g., 15 million children and adolescents are exposed to environmental tobacco smoke in the home[43]), or in some instances, estimates based on attributable risk (e.g., more than 400,000 deaths result from cigarette smoking in the United States each year[44]).

Lists and rankings are also simple but powerful approaches for data presentation. Such lists resonate well in American society,[20] and they are commonly used in non-health contexts. For audiences with low numeracy, rankings without numbers (e.g., the 3 major risk factors for a health condition) may be appropriate.[2,45] Presenting rankings of numbers in terciles or quartiles (to minimize misperceptions based on small differences) may be used with more mathematically sophisticated audiences.

When possible, simple visuals should be used to communicate data that cannot be adequately summarized in a few numbers or as a list or ranking. Both the general public and news media representatives generally prefer and understand pie charts. Maps, pie charts, and trend lines are likely to be understood by the news media, administrators, elected officials, and persons in voluntary or private health organizations. Bar charts are often well-understood by policy makers and other selected nonscientific audiences.

CHALLENGES AND BARRIERS

PRESENTING TOO MUCH DATA

Presenting too much data, or data overload, is probably the most common problem when communicating with nonscientists.[31] Overload occurs because public health professionals believe that audiences share their interest in data; believe that having more data indicates more knowledge (or will prevent criticism); or believe that more data will justify the analytic approach, results, or conclusions. Using too much data is counterproductive for nonscientific audiences, since most lay people can comprehend only a few key pieces of information (chapter 4). Data should thus be used sparingly and for a specific purpose. Presenting tables of data should especially be avoided because this quickly leads to overload.

DESCRIBING METHODOLOGY

In contrast to scientific audiences, nonscientific audiences rarely want or need to know about the methodology or the strengths and weaknesses of data analyses. Most nonscientists will respect the public health practitioner's background and position of authority, and will assume the information is credible. Discussion of data quality and methodology may not be understood by many nonscientific audiences, nor are general audiences likely to be interested in these issues. There are a few exceptions to this recommendation. Quality and methodology are likely to be challenged in adversarial situations,[31] in some risk communication situations, or when synthetic data estimates or projections are used in policy deliberations.

USING STATISTICAL TERMS

Statistical terminology should be avoided. Measures designed to determine whether the observed differences are the result of chance (i.e., p-values, 95% confidence limits), although important for analyzing data, should not be part of the communication with nonscientific audiences. The one exception is that news media representatives commonly report 95% confidence limits as the margin of error or the accuracy of a survey (e.g., within 3 percent). The phrase "statistically significant" rarely is meaningful to these audiences, nor are terms such as "incidence," "prevalence," "regression analysis," or "correlation coefficient."

SUMMARY

Communicating public health data to nonscientists is challenging. With the advent of the Internet, there are more data and other scientific information available, but certain publications such as *Health, United States* and the *Statistical Abstract* remain valuable resources. Before communicating, it is essential to assess the quality and interpretation of the science, as well as the credibility, credentials, and potential conflicts of interest of those who report the information. General considerations when translating data to nonscientists include presenting data ethically, being selective in the choice of data, considering the type of data that would be of interest to the audience (e.g., magnitude, context, and meaning), simplifying and explaining unfamiliar terms and concepts, and creating numeric analogies.

Actual numbers, simple lists, rankings, and visuals are the recommended formats for communicating quantitative information to nonscientists. Data overload, discussing methodologic issues, and attempting to explain statistical uncertainty are common problems.

With the plethora of information now available, the great interest in health among nonscientists, and low numeracy among many audiences, locating and translating public health data will become increasingly important for public health practitioners.

CHAPTER 3 ENDNOTES

1. Beck EM, ed. *Bartlett's Familiar Quotations.* 15th ed. Boston: Little, Brown & Company; 1980:80.
2. Paulos JA. *Innumeracy: Mathematical Illiteracy and its Consequences.* New York: Vintage Books; 1990.
3. Slovic P. Perception of risk. *Science.* 1987;236:280-285.
4. Bernier RH, Watson VM, Nowell A, Emery B, St. Pierre J, eds. *EpiSource: a Guide to Resources in Epidemiology.* Roswell, GA: The Epidemiology Monitor; 1998.
5. Humphreys BL, Ruffin AB, Cahn MA, Rambo N. Powerful connections for public health: the National Library of Medicine and the National Network of Libraries of Medicine. *Am J Public Health.*1999;89:1633-1636.
6. Shipman JP. Document delivery suppliers. Richmond, VA: Virginia Commonwealth University, Tomkins-McCaw library for the health sciences. Web site address: http://www.library.vcu.edu/tml/docsupp.
7. National Library of Medicine's Locator Plus. Web site address: http://locatorplus.gov/.
8. National Center for Health Statistics. *Health, United States, 2001 With Urban and Rural Health Chartbook.* Hyattsville, Maryland: National Center for Health Statistics; 2001.
9. *Statistical Abstract of the United States: 2001.* Washington, DC: U.S. Census Bureau, 2001.
10. Youth Risk Behavioral Surveillance System Web site address: http://www.cdc.gov/nccdphp/dash/yrbs.
11. National Center for Health Statistics. Web site address: http://www.cdc.gov/nchs.
12. Behavioral Risk Factor Surveillance System Web site. Web site address: http://www.cdc.gov/brfss.
13. Agency for Healthcare Quality Research. Web site address: http://www.ahrq.gov.
14. U.S. Census Bureau. Web site address: http://www.census.gov.
15. Maxwell B. *How to Find Information on the Internet.* Washington, DC: Congressional Quarterly Inc.; 1998.
16. Berland GK, Elliott MN, Morales LS, et al. Health information on the Internet—Accessibility, quality, and readability in English and Spanish. *JAMA.* 2001;285:2612-2621.
17. Savitz DA, Harris RP, Brownson RC. *Methods in Chronic Disease Epidemiology.* In: *Chronic Disease Epidemiology and Control.* 2nd ed. Washington, DC: American Public Health Association; 1998:27-54.
18. Riegelman RK. *Studying a Study and Testing a Test,* 4th ed. Philadelphia, PA: Lippincott Williams & Wilkins, 2000.
19. Cohn V, , Cope L. *News & Numbers: A Guide to Reporting Statistical Claims and Controversies in Health and Other Fields.* 2nd ed. Ames, IA: Iowa State University Press; 2001.
20. Paulos JA. *A Mathematician Reads the Newspaper.* New York: Basic Books; 1995.
21. Schwartz LM, Woloshin S. Marketing medicine to the public: a reader's guide. *JAMA* 2002;287:774-775.
22. Huff D, Geiss I. *How to Lie with Statistics.* New York: WW Norton & Company; 1993.
23. Harvard Center for Risk Analysis. *Risk in Perspective.* Health Insight: A Consumer Guide to Taking Charge of Health Information. Vol 7. Boston, MA; Harvard Center for Risk Analysis; October 1999.
24. Coughlin S, Beachamp TL. *Ethics and Epidemiology.* New York: Oxford; 1996.
25. Maier MH. *The Data Game: Controversies in Social Science Statistics.* 2nd ed. Armonk, NY: Sharpe; 1995.
26. Tufte ER. *The Visual Display of Quantitative Information.* Cheshire, CT: Graphics Press; 1983.

27. Templeton M, Fitzgerald SS. *Schaum's Quick Guide to Great Presentation Skills.* New York: McGraw-Hill; 1999.
28. Gastel B. *Presenting Science to the Public.* Philadelphia, PA: ISI Press; 1983.
29. Gastel B. *Health Writer's Handbook.* Ames, IA: Iowa State University Press; 1997.
30. Witte, K. The manipulative nature of health communication research. *Am Behav Scientist.* 1994;38:285-293
31. Wallack L, Dorfman L, Jernigan D, Themba M. *Media Advocacy and Public Health. Power for Prevention.* Newbury Park, CA: Sage Publications; 1993.
32. Centers for Disease Control and Prevention. Measles—United States, first 26 weeks, 1993. *MMWR.* 1993;42:813-816.
33. Lipkus IM, Samsa G, Rimer BK. General performance on a numeracy scale among highly educated samples. *Med Decis Making.* 2001;21:37-44.
34. Woloshin S, Schwartz LM, Moncur M, Gabriel S, Tosteson AN. Assessing values for health: numeracy matters. *Med Decis Making.* 2001;21:382-90.
35. Last JM (ed). *A Dictionary of Epidemiology.* 3rd ed. New York: Oxford; 1995.
36. U.S. Department of Health and Human Services. *Media Strategies for Smoking Control: Guidelines.* Bethesda, MD: National Institutes of Health; 1989. NIH Pub. No. 89-3013.
37. Gigerenzer G. The psychology of good judgment: frequency formats and simple algorithms. *Medical Decision Making.* 1996;16:270-280.
38. Advocacy Institute. *By the Numbers: A Guide to the Tactical Use of Statistics for Positive Policy Change.* Washington, DC: Advocacy Institute, Blowing Smoke Advisory No.2.
39. National Research Council. *Understanding Risk: Informing Decisions in a Democratic Society.* Washington, DC: National Academy Press; 1996.
40. Wallack L, Woodruff K, Dorfman L, Diaz I. *News for a Change: An Advocate's Guide to Working with the Media.* Thousand Oaks, CA: Sage; 1999.
41. Brain B. *Weapons for Temperance Warfare: Some Plans and Programs.* Boston, MA: United Society of Christian Endeavor; 1897.
42. Pertschuk M, Wilbur P. *Media Advocacy: Reframing Public Debate.* Washington, DC: Benton Foundation and the Center for Strategic Communications; 1991.
43. Centers for Disease Control and Prevention. State-specific prevalence of cigarette smoking among adults, and children's and adolescents' exposure to environmental tobacco smoke—United States, 1996. *MMWR.* 1997;46:1038-1043.
44. Nelson DE, Kirkendall RS, Lawton RL, et al. State estimates of smoking-attributable mortality and years of potential life lost, 1990. *MMWR CDC Surveillance Summary.* 1994;43(SS-1):1-8.
45. Root J, Stableford S. *Write It Easy-to-Read: A Guide to Creating Plain English Materials.* Biddleford ME: Maine AHEC Health Literacy Center; 1997.

SUGGESTED READINGS

Cohn V., Cope L. *News & Numbers: A Guide to Reporting Statistical Claims and Controversies in Health and Other Fields, 2nd Edition.* Ames, IA: Iowa State University Press, 2001.

Gastel B. *Health Writer's Handbook.* Ames, IA: Iowa State University Press, 1997.

Paulos, JA. *A Mathematician Reads the Newspaper.* New York: Basic Books, 1995.

Riegelman RK. *Studying a Study and Testing a Test,* 4th ed. Philadelphia, PA: Lippincott, Williams & Wilkins, 2000.

Wallack L., Dorfman L., Jernagin D., Themba M. *Media Advocacy and Public Health.* Newbury Park, CA: Sage, 1993.

Wallack L., Woodruff K., Dorfman L., Diaz I., *News for a Change: An Advocate's Guide to Working with the Media.* Thousand Oaks, CA: Sage, 19998.

PART II:

AUDIENCES

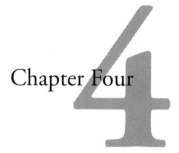

Chapter Four

GENERAL PUBLIC: COMMUNICATING TO INFORM

Max Lum, EdD
Claudia Parvanta, PhD
Ed Maibach, PhD
Elaine Arkin
David E. Nelson, MD, MPH

One of the 10 essential public health services is to "inform, educate, and empower people about health issues."[1] Accurate health information must be provided to people to make appropriate choices to improve their health. An enumeration of the federal, state and territorial workforce indicated that in 2000, about one per cent of individuals were classified as "health educator" or "public relations/media specialist."[2] However, the ability to communicate scientific information is included as a core competency for nearly every level of public health staff across all essential services.[1]

There is an extensive body of research on communicating with the general public.[3-9] Such communication covers a spectrum that ranges from providing information to facilitate informed decision-making, to providing information to persuade people to make changes; for example, thoroughly cooking meat before serving. Because of the differences between these communication purposes, and because of the vast knowledge base, the topic of communication with the general public has been divided into two chapters.

This chapter covers topics critical to facilitating informed decision-making, including audience factors (segmentation, literacy, numeracy, culture, language, and preferred communication channels), information processing, and message development. Chapter 5 presents information on making communication more persuasive in order to facilitate health behavior change. (Readers are strongly encouraged to read chapters 4 and 5 in sequence.)

The distinction between communicating to inform versus communicating to persuade is somewhat artificial. Information and persuasion may be combined in one message: "Trends in alcohol use among pregnant women are increasing—don't drink if you are pregnant."[10] It has been argued that there is an element of persuasion in all health communication.[11]

BACKGROUND

Communication to inform the general public ranges from one-on-one conversations to national or international media campaigns. It can be done proactively or reactively (i.e., in response to requests from the public for information). Examples of proactively communicating to inform the general public include: raising awareness of a new or acute health problem, helping to reduce fear in an emergency, raising or maintaining interest in an ongoing health problem, reporting health trends, and facilitating informed decision-making. The types of public health issues of which practitioners inform general public audiences are numerous; they include issues such as emerging infectious diseases, trends in youth smoking, and benefits and risks of mammography screening for women aged 40-49 years. Persuading the general public, as discussed in the next chapter, involves recommending that audiences take specific actions such as smoking cessation or using condoms.

There are many instances, however, when communicating to inform general public audiences is the main emphasis. Box 4.1 is a specific example of this type of communication.

BOX 4.1

The director of the state cancer control program has been asked by the statewide cancer coalition to develop prostate cancer screening materials for men who attend public clinics. After reviewing the scientific literature, the program director concludes that there is no consensus about the efficacy of prostate-specific antigen (PSA) testing: some organizations recommend periodic screening of men aged 50 years and older and other organizations do not.[12] The director has staff members develop an easy-to-read one-page fact sheet that briefly describes the PSA controversy and the pros and cons of PSA testing. Health care providers at the clinics are instructed to review the fact sheet with each patient, answer questions, and to allow each individual to make his own decision about testing.

Communicating health information to the public must be a two-way process in which practitioners work with, and listen carefully to, their audience. Too often health education materials such as pamphlets, oral presentations, videos, and media spots are based on the mistaken belief that communication consists of professionals sending a container of information through a conduit and that audience members remove ideas from the container.[13] Audience input is essential so that communicators can adjust their messages and channels to more effectively reach intended audiences. It is essential to recognize that meaning arises only when listeners, readers, or viewers actively make sense of what they hear, read, or see. Meaning is not transmitted by experts so much as it is constructed by listeners.

Successfully communicating to inform is guided by two primary requirements: (1) determining needs, and (2) providing what is needed. Needs assessment includes discovering the perceived health information needs, knowledge, opinions, attitudes, cultural factors, and preferred information formats of the nonscientist audience. Providing what is needed requires shaping technical information and supporting data in a way that it can be understood and used by the lay audience. The ideal outcome of communicating to inform is that the audience, being fully confident that the information they receive is accurate, engages in effective decision-making. Their values, comfort level with risk or uncertainty, and other factors might shape the choice they eventually make, but the information has empowered them to choose wisely.

Presenting unbiased information to assist decision-making is not equivalent to handing out data tables. Work must be done to present information so that it is inviting and easy to understand. Below are some of the key concepts and tools that facilitate this process.

GETTING TO KNOW THE AUDIENCE

The term "general public" is actually misleading, as there are few times when the entire public can be addressed with the same message in the same manner. Public audiences need to be divided into groups, or segmented, and their needs in terms of literacy, understanding of numerical information (numeracy), cultural issues, foreign language use, and communication channels must be determined.

AUDIENCE SEGMENTATION

This topic was introduced in chapter 2. Dividing larger populations into smaller, homogeneous groups is essential for communicating efficiently. Proactive health communication allows health practitioners to target messages toward populations of greatest interest; for example focusing childhood immunization messages on parents and other child-care providers. This helps prevent wasting resources on populations who have no interest or need for the information. Segmentation also facilitates delivery of public health information in reactive situations such as epidemics, cluster investigations, or acute environmental exposures. Approaches commonly used to segment the general public include sociodemographics, behavioral, psychobehavioral, and multivariate methods.[14–19]

The amount of time and resources devoted to audience segmentation varies by situation. If a practitioner is reacting to a request for information from a member of the public in a one-on-one interaction, then segmentation is clearly unnecessary. However, segmentation is applicable and invaluable in most situations where practitioners are developing materials for multiple purposes, such as oral presentations, written materials, or communication through the mass media or Internet Web sites.

At a minimum, practitioners should segment audiences by educational or reading level and try to ascertain if there are reasons to use a finer segmentation strategy (e.g., existing knowledge, opinions, attitudes, or cultural factors). For larger public communication efforts, more extensive segmentation efforts based on behavioral, psychobehavioral, or multivariate (methods or some combination will probably be needed.

PRIMARY, SECONDARY AND TERTIARY AUDIENCES

The concept of primary, secondary and tertiary audiences was also introduced in chapter 2. The key user of information is generally considered the primary audience, but health practitioners often work through intermediaries to provide information to the user, either through individuals in direct contact (secondary audiences), or through individuals and organizations with indirect contact (tertiary audiences). Separate packets of information can be developed for health care providers, news media representatives, elected officials, community groups, churches, businesses, unions, voluntary health organizations, and private health organizations.

Secondary and tertiary audiences are important because the public is far more likely to be exposed to, attend to, and believe messages from these familiar sources than from unknown public health officials. In many (if not most) situations, practitioners use secondary and tertiary audiences because doing so is usually more efficient and effective. For example, informing the public about the potential adverse health effects of using space heaters in poorly ventilated rooms will be more effective if health care providers, the news media, and retail outlets are notified and asked to share this information with the general public.

LITERACY AND NUMERACY

A major concern for developing informational messages for the public is low literacy and numeracy. According to a national adult literacy survey, about 90 million American adults (47% of the U.S. population) demonstrate low levels of literacy, that is, they read at or below about an 8th grade level.[20,21] Individuals with impaired literacy often experience great difficulty with the writing, computation, and processing skills necessary to understand and make informed decisions about their health.

Most Americans have a limited understanding of basic science concepts;[22] technical and medical terminologies, and the dynamic nature of the scientific method, are poorly understood. Many people overestimate what science can accomplish. Although almost half of Americans are very confident in the leadership of the scientific and medical communities, only one in nine Americans feels well-informed about science and technology. One survey found that only one American in four can provide some of the reasons for the thinning of the ozone layer, and fewer than one in ten can describe the meaning of the word "molecule".[22]

Many Americans also have problems with math literacy, also referred to as numeracy.[23] Unfortunately, this means that many members of the general public do not understand basic mathematical concepts commonly used in public health such as rates, probabilities, frequencies, and percentages.[23,24]

Low reading levels, a poor understanding of science, and low numeracy ability all have important implications for communicating with the general public. Practitioners must simplify public health information for these audiences. Scientific concepts and technical terms must be introduced slowly and explained clearly and carefully. Great care must be taken when developing messages that contain potentially complex numbers. For example, the problems inherent in discussing probability can sometimes be addressed by using qualitative expressions such as "likely" or "highly probable," but such terms are understood to mean different things to different people. These issues are discussed more fully in chapters 3 and 13.

CULTURE AND LANGUAGE

The population of the United States is becoming more diverse, with an increasing percentage of the population of Hispanic origin, and a growth in immigration from many continents.[25] This diversity creates new challenges for developing informational public health messages.[26-28] Common English language terms may not translate well; "feeling blue" may not be meaningful in other cultures. Conversely, phrases from other cultures may not translate easily into mainstream American culture. For instance, Latinos may talk about "*susto*," which is an illness believed to arise from fright.[27] There are also important language differences within given cultural groups such as Mexican-Americans, Puerto Ricans, or Cuban-Americans. This must be considered when translating across languages, as the same word in Spanish may have different meanings to each of these Latino subgroups.

If the target population includes individuals from different cultures or individuals who speak different languages, public health communication messages must be tailored accordingly.[26-28] Again, this requires a thorough understanding of the audience. For example, if visuals are used, drawings or photographs of individuals from the same ethnic group as the targeted audience may be helpful.[4,9,26] If English language messages are translated, the translator should be fluent with the dialect of the target population (e.g., if the target population is of Puerto Rican descent, then the translator should be familiar with Puerto Rican Spanish).

Working directly with populations that use English as a second language to gather input before developing informational materials is more effective than translating English language materials into foreign languages. These materials can be "back-translated" to ensure the meaning is equivalent, but not necessarily a literal, translation of English.

PREFERRED COMMUNICATION CHANNELS

Communication channels, like channels on a television set, are the "places" (virtual or real) where people receive information. Channels are often referred to as the "where" of health communication. Channel choices are expanding, with new options in electronic, print, mass media, community, and interpersonal outlets. Health communication planners strive for efficiencies and convergence in media channels to minimize the amount of creative development time and money required to disseminate information.

Large-scale mass media—city-wide newspapers, national magazines, national television—are generally the least sensitive channels to target messages to specific populations. However, within communities, local television affiliates, outdoor advertising (billboards, bus placards), and radio can be used to carry targeted messages to particular groups. Direct mail items can be sent to specific census block codes that can be cross-referenced with other data bases that provide information on language choice, socioeconomic level or other relevant information about the intended recipients.

The entertainment and advertising aspects of mass media are also a means of informing the public about public health topics.[29,30] Examples include story lines in television shows, paid advertising, and public service announcements (PSAs). Many public health programs use the mass media in proactive communication efforts to reach the public for both informational and persuasive purposes. Developing informational public health messages for mass media campaigns is a complex task that is beyond the scope of this book. (Readers are referred to references 6, 14, 29, and 30 for further discussion.)

Communication channel decisions affect whether the intended audience ever sees or hears the information. For example, while Internet use is expanding in the United States, it is far from universal. Presenting information through donated public service announcement time slots on television usually restricts the airing to late night or early morning hours when few of the targeted audience may be watching. Unless special events are heavily promoted, requiring large investments of time or money, information about them will not reach a large number of persons in any community. Consultation with professional media specialists can help public health practitioners bundle the right combination of communication channels to reach any audiences.

INFORMATION PROCESSING

Perhaps the most fundamental fact for understanding the communication process is that people are limited in how much information they can process.[31,32] To cope with information processing limitations, individuals selectively choose information based on its apparent value and their own biases; they simplify the information and look for shortcuts to help them rapidly reach a conclusion or make a decision. Audience members inevitably simplify complex information, so the role of public health practitioners is to help them simplify this information appropriately.[32,33]

Glanz et al[8] have summarized the communication implications of information processing theory. First, to overcome people's limited information processing capacity, choose the most important and useful points to communicate. Second, to overcome limitations in people's information searching processes, provide information that takes little effort to obtain, is attention-getting, and is clear. Third, to work within people's comfort zones, synthesize key information so that it has meaning and appeal to audience members.

An audience's level of involvement with the specific issue is a critical variable in determining how they will subsequently process information on the issue. The Elaboration Likelihood Model (ELM)[34] suggests that people at high levels of issue involvement will process information carefully, with an eye toward examining the merits of the communicator's arguments (for instance, persons who have coronary artery disease are likely to pay attention to messages about recognizing the signs and symptoms of a heart attack). Conversely, people at low levels of issue involvement tend to process information only superficially, looking for overt cues as to whether the message applies to them. These cues can include attributes of the communicator (e.g., appearance), the source of information (e.g., expertise), or endorsements by respected individuals or organizations. Communicators with a perceived self-interest, such as, a corporate spokesperson, are often not trusted, even if they are perceived to be experts in their fields. In some situations, especially where there are polarized positions or emotions are high, public health professionals may need to reinforce that they are acting out of a concern for the community's health and not out of self-interest.

When communicating with low involvement audiences, it is not productive to include much specific information, as these audiences are unlikely to attend to such messages. Instead, practitioners should consider increasing the emotional content or use anecdotal evidence to get the attention of the target audience.[35] An example of this occurred in a radio public service announcement targeted at young workers in noisy workplaces as the service announcement contained sounds of children playing and laughing. The message for young workers was to protect their hearing to prevent noise-induced hearing loss so, as they age, they would be able to experience the sounds of their grandchildren.

How people understand and process information about uncertainty, probability, and risk is another important consideration. People pay more attention to information that is proven and reliable over information that is thought to be uncertain.[36] For instance, men who believe they are not at risk for HIV may best be reached by including specific examples showing that they are at increased risk based on expert medical opinion.[37] Among certain audiences, presentations that include uncertainties tend to create suspicion about the source ("Why don't they just tell me—what are they hiding?"). These audiences lay blame on others for the cause of the problem or discount the risk to themselves.[38] The preference of audiences for "information certainty" presents a challenge to communicators because most public health data have an inherent element of uncertainty.

MESSAGE DEVELOPMENT AND PLANNING

Table 4.1 lists recommendations for developing and planning information messages for the public.[39] New messages developed for health-related topics must avoid cliches, otherwise audiences may tune them out. New communication channels, or new uses for existing channels, should be considered when feasible. A simple but powerful technique for messages is to ask the audience to pay attention; closely related is the need to personalize the message, explaining the issue as if speaking directly to one individual. Rather than using ill-defined words such as somewhere or sometime, describe the here and now. Also, qualifying words such as "may be likely to" should be avoided.

TABLE 4.1—RECOMMENDATIONS FOR MESSAGE DEVELOPMENT AND PLANNING

Develop new messages and ways to use communication channels

Ask the audience to pay attention to the message

Personalize the message to the intended recipient

Talk about the here and now, not "somewhere" or "sometime"

Avoid use of qualifiers such as "may be likely to"

Use a simple and direct message

Consider using irony

Pre-test message with audience

Surprise audience by placing messages in unexpected places

Adapted from Reference 39

As mentioned in the previous section, messages need to be simple and clear to be readily understood by audiences; avoid confusing or difficult language.[5,40] In some situations, irony can be used to gain attention and deliver the message. Messages should always be pre-tested with audience. Finally, consider ways to surprise audiences by placing messages in unexpected places (e.g. posting sunburn prevention messages at swimming club dressing rooms, water quality information in bait shops, and nutrition information in bookstores).

PRE-TESTING

The importance of pre-testing materials for general public audiences cannot be overestimated. Pre-testing not only helps improve the message, but it provides insights into visuals, recognition of important secondary audiences, communication channels, and context.[41] Five examples from the National Clearinghouse for Alcohol and Drug Information described in Box 4.2 illustrate the role of pre-testing in development and planning, such as recognizing mixed messages, assessing the acceptability of messages, increasing audience involvement, determining personal relevance, and gauging sensitive or controversial elements.[41]

BOX 4.2

In an effort to reduce underage drinking, the initial message was: "Part of growing up is learning how to make wise decisions. If you choose to drink, drink responsibly. Don't overdo it and don't drink and drive." Pre-testing with the intended audience demonstrated that this was an unclear (mixed) message. After testing, the message was changed to: "Part of growing up is learning how to make wise decisions. You should know that if you choose to drink before you are 21, you are breaking the law."

During focus groups to develop materials for children concerning tobacco, drug and alcohol abuse, several students mentioned the importance of selecting age-appropriate language. Several children mentioned that the phrase ". . . alcohol and other drugs make you feel clumsy" was confusing. Better words suggested by the children included "dizzy" or "confused."

One program found that when pre-testing an educational comic book, children in focus groups enjoyed acting out the parts. The result was a new idea: a play about alcohol, tobacco, and other drugs for elementary school students.

The National PTA learned through focus group sessions that parents rarely or never seek out information about alcohol, tobacco and drug abuse. Consequently, direct distribution of materials was considered important. Moreover, parents identified the need for practical ideas for dealing with difficult situations. This later finding resulted in a new program providing them with practical, hands-on skills training.

Would a televised demonstration of breast self-examination on a live model be an affront to viewers? Pre-test results of such a PSA indicated that respondents held a range of views about the propriety of this demonstration.

CHALLENGES AND BARRIERS

MINIMAL INTEREST IN INFORMATION

Except in acute situations, getting general public audiences to pay attention to public health information is the largest challenge to communication, especially if audiences have a low level of involvement with an issue.[34] This can be a special problem for long-standing chronic health issues such as alcohol abuse or smoking; the problem underscores the importance of personalizing messages, stressing the relevance of the information, and working with secondary or tertiary audiences such as health care providers or community organizations.

CROWDED INFORMATION ENVIRONMENT

Closely related to general public audiences' lack of attention or indifference to health messages is the problem of the crowded information environment. On an almost daily basis, individuals in the United States are exposed to hundreds of messages from multiple sources. These messages seek to gain the attention of the public on many different topics or issues, ranging from advertising for automobiles or pharmaceutical products to raising awareness about global warming. Because the "message marketplace" for the general public is so crowded, it commonly leads to overload, thus necessitating the development of public health messages that grab the attention of intended audiences.

FAILURE TO SEE NEED FOR DATA OR DISBELIEF OF SCIENTIFIC FINDINGS

Audiences may perceive that scientific data or information from research studies are trivial, unnecessary, or are "wrong" compared to their personal observations or existing beliefs.

For example, residents in one Florida metropolitan county were concerned about background radiation releases and believed that their county had the highest cancer death rate in the Florida. Attempts to explain the problems of using all-cancer mortality data and of failing to age-adjust data were unsuccessful. Use of a simple visual chart that compared cancer mortality and morbidity data by county helped to address the confusion among the residents. However, in many situations, merely presenting data and other information to counter existing beliefs is unsuccessful. More work is then needed to gain the trust of the community and to involve community members in presenting the information (chapter 13). A recognizable trusted presenter may be more successful in reaching the target audience than an unknown public health official.

UNCERTAINTY OF INFORMATION

Scientific data and existing scientific theories have some level of uncertainty. The very nature of scientific inquiry means that beliefs may be disproved (the role of diet in peptic ulcer disease, for example). Given that people value certainty over uncertainty, it can be difficult to convince the general public of the importance of an informational message. So, except in certain situations (e.g., risk communication), the uncertainty should be minimized when communicating to inform general public audiences.

SUMMARY

Communicating to the general public is a two-way process, as meaning is not transmitted by experts as much as it is constructed by listeners. Audience segmentation is critical for identifying and targeting specific populations and for maximizing the use of resources. Secondary and tertiary audiences such as health care providers, news media, and community groups are commonly used to reach the general population. Other important audience considerations include literacy, numeracy, language, culture, and preferred communication channels.

Information processing theory suggests that individuals have a limited capacity to attend to and process information. Messages must cover the key points, should reach audiences with minimal effort, be simple and clear, and be meaningful and appealing. Message development and planning recommendations include personalizing content, asking audiences to pay attention, using simple language, and, when appropriate, using irony. Pre-testing messages with the intended audience is critical, especially for proactive communication, as it can help improve the message, the learning context, and the dissemination plan; and it can eliminate embarrassment.

The future of communicating to inform the general public requires increased attention to the two-way nature of such communication and the need to engage these audiences in the process. The increased use of the Internet, along with continued news media interest, will increase the availability of and the demand for health information by the public.

CHAPTER 4 ENDNOTES

1. Council on Linkages Between Academia & Public Health. *Core Competencies for Public Health*. April 2001. Available at:http:/www.trainingfinder.org (last accessed: 6/4/02)
2. Gebbie K. *The Public Health Work Force. Enumeration 2000*. Health Resources and Services Administration; Rockville, MD: 2000.

3. Bradac JJ, ed. *Message Effects in Communication Science*. Newbury Park, CA: Sage Publications; 1989.
4. Niteke S, Shaw A. Developing materials for low-income low-literate audiences. *J Nutr Educ.* 1980;18:226-236.
6. Hornik R, ed. *Public Health Communication: Evidence for Behavior Change*. Mahwah, NJ: Erlbaum, 2002.
7. Wallack L. *Media Advocacy and Public Health*. Newbury Park, CA: Sage, 1993.
8. Glanz K, Lewis FM, Rimer BK eds. *Health Behavior and Health Education: Theory, Research, and Practice. 2nd ed.* San Francisco, CA: Jossey-Bass; 1997.
9. Valente TW. *Evaluating Health Promotion Programs*. New York: Oxford; 2002.
10. U.S. Department of Health and Human Services. *Making Health Communication Programs Work: A Planner's Guide*. Bethesda, MD: U.S. Department of Health and Human Services, National Institutes of Health, National Cancer Institute; 1992: NIH publication 92-1493. Available at: http://oc.nci.nih.gov/services/HCPW/HOME.HTM.
11. Witte K. Preventing AIDS through persuasive communications: a framework for constructing effective, culturally-specific, preventive health messages. *International Intercultural Communication Annual.* 1992;16:67-86.
12. U.S. Preventive Services Task Force. *Guide to Clinical Preventive Services*. Baltimore, MD: Williams and Wilkins; 1996.
13. Reddy MJ. The conduit metaphor: a case of frame conflict in our language about language. In: Oktony A, ed. *Metaphor and Thought*. Cambridge, U.K.: Cambridge University Press; 1979.
14. Maibach E, Parrott R, eds. *Designing Health Messages: Approaches from Communication Theory and Practice*. Thousand Oaks, CA: Sage; 1995.
15. Slater MD. Choosing audience segmentation strategies and methods for health communication. In: Maibach E, and Parrott R, eds. *Designing Health Messages: Approaches from Communication Theory and Practice*. Thousand Oaks, CA: Sage, 1995: 186-198.
16. Weinstein A. *Market Segmentation*. Chicago: Probus, 1994.
17. Bandura A. *Social Foundations of Thought and Action: A Social Cognitive Theory.* Englewood Cliffs: NJ: Prentice Hall; 1986.
18. Bandura A. *Self-Efficacy: The Exercise of Control*. New York: W.H. Freeman; 1997.
19. Prochaska JO, DiClemente CC, Norcross JC. In search of how people change: applications to the addictive behaviors. *Am Psychologist.* 1992;47:1102-1114.
20. Root J, Stableford S. *Write It Easy-to-Read. A Guide to Creating Plain English Materials*. Biddleford, ME: Maine; AHEC Literacy Center, 1997.
21. Kirsch I, Jungeblut A, Jerkins L, Kolstad A. *Adult Literacy in America*. Princeton: NJ: Educational Testing Service; 1993.
22. National Science Board. *Science and Engineering Indicators 2000*. Washington, DC: National Science Foundation; 2000.
23. Paulos, J. *Innumeracy: Mathematical Illiteracy and its Consequences*. New York: Vintage Books; 1990.
24. Gilovich T, Vallone T, Tversky A. The hot hand in basketball: On the misperception of random sequences. *Cognitive Psychol.* 1985;17:295-314.
25. U.S. Bureau of the Census. *Statistical Abstract of the United States: 2001*. Washington, DC: U.S. Census Bureau; 2001.
26. Centers for Disease Control and Prevention. *Simply Put: Tips for Creating Easy-To-Read Print Materials Your Audience Will Want to Read and Use*. 2nd edition. Atlanta, GA: Centers for Disease Control and Prevention, Office of Communication, 1999.
27. Rigoglioso RL. Multiculturalism in practice. *The Picker Report.* 1995;3:1,12-13.
28. Gudykunst WB, Mody B. *Handbook of International and Intercultural Communication,* 2nd ed. Thousand Oaks, CA: Sage; 2002.
29. Atkin C, Wallack L, eds. *Mass Communication and Public Health: Complexities and Conflicts*. Newbury Park, CA: Sage; 1990.
30. Rice RE, Atkins CK, eds. *Public Communication Campaigns,* 2nd ed. Newbury Park, CA: Sage, 1989: 131-150.
31. Bettman J. *An Information Processing Theory of Consumer Choice*. Reading, Mass.: Addison Wesley; 1979.

32. National Academy of Sciences. *Improving Risk Communication.* Washington, DC: National Academy of Sciences; 1989.
33. Holtgrave DR, Tinsley BJ, Kay LS. Encouraging risk reduction: a decision-making approach to message design. In: Maibach E & Parrott R, eds. *Designing Health Messages.* Thousand Oaks, CA: Sage Publications, 1995.
34. Petty RE, Cacioppo JT. The elaboration likelihood model of persuasion. *Advances in Experimental and Social Psychology.* 1986;19:123-205.
35. Flora J, Maibach E, Maccoby N. The role of media across four levels of health promotion intervention. *Annual Review of Public Health.* Palo Alto: Annual Reviews Inc; 1989.
36. Slovic P. Informing and educating the public about risk. *Risk Anal.* 1986;6:403-415.
37. Marin G. AIDS prevention among Hispanics: needs, risk behaviors, and cultural values. *Pub Health Rep.* 1989;104:411-415.
38. Navarro M. AIDS in Hispanic community: threat ignored. *New York Times,* December 29, 1989; B1, B10.
39. Parrot RL. Motivation to attend to health messages. Presentation of content and linguistic considerations. In: Maibach E, Parrott RL, eds. *Designing Health Messages.* Thousand Oaks, CA: Sage; 1995:7-23.
40. Mayer RE. What have we learned about increasing the meaningfulness of science prose? *Science Educ.* 1983;67:223-237.
41. National Clearinghouse for Alcohol and Drug Information. *Technical Assistance Bulletin: You Can Manage Focus Groups Effectively for Maximum Impact.* Rockville, MD: Center for Substance Abuse Prevention, 1994. Available at: http://www.health.org.

SUGGESTED READINGS AND RESOURCES

Glanz K, Lewis FM, Rimer BK, eds. Health Behavior and Health Education: Theory, Research, and Practice. 2nd ed. San Francisco, CA: Jossey-Bass; 1997.

Parrot RL. Motivation to attend to health messages. Presentation of content and linguistic considerations. In: Maibach E, Parrott RL, eds. *Designing Health Messages.* Thousand Oaks, CA: Sage; 1995: 7-23.

Slater MD. Choosing audience segmentation strategies and methods for health communication. In: Maibach E, and Parrott R, eds. *Designing Health Messages: Approaches from Communication Theory and Practice.* Thousand Oaks, CA: Sage; 1995: 186-198.

Substance Abuse and Mental Health Services Administration, National Clearinghouse for Alcohol and Drug Information. *Technical Assistance Bulletin: You Can Manage Focus Groups Effectively for Maximum Impact.* Rockville, MD: Center for Substance Abuse Prevention, 1994. Available at: http://www.health.org.

U.S. Department of Health and Human Services. *Making Health Communication Programs Work: A Planner's Guide.* Bethesda, MD: U.S. Department of Health and Human Services, National Institutes of Health, National Cancer Institute; 1992: NIH publication 92-1493. Available at: http://oc.nci.nih.gov/services/hpcw/home.htm.

Chapter Five

GENERAL PUBLIC: COMMUNICATING TO PERSUADE

Elaine Arkin
Edward Maibach, PhD
Claudia Parvanta, PhD

As introduced in chapter 2, planning for public health communication depends on whether the primary purpose is to inform audiences to facilitate decision-making or to persuade audiences. Persuasion refers to using information to help change opinions, attitudes, or behaviors, and it is probably the most common purpose for communication in public health practice. Examples of persuasion in public health are legion, such as encouraging smoking prevention and cessation, condom use, early prenatal care, prevention of driving under the influence of drugs or alcohol, or persuading parents to immunize their young children.

Chapter 4 provided an overview of strategies and tactics when the primary purpose is to inform the general public. This chapter adds additional tools for communicating persuasively; it includes an overview of behavior change communication, persuasion and other commonly used theories, recommendations for understanding general public audiences, and recommendations for developing and delivering messages. Although most of the material presented in this chapter is based on large-scale interventions and mass communication, the principles and recommendations are directly applicable to less formal persuasive communication situations common to public health practice.

BACKGROUND

Public health practitioners have a number of choices of how to persuade people to make changes, and each is based on theories and perspectives. Rothschild has described a framework in which education, marketing, and law represent a spectrum of approaches to prompt socially responsible behavior.[1] Although his description is much more complex, it centers on individual decision-making and the perceived costs and benefits of any proposed new behavior, idea, or product.

Figure 5.1 illustrates this relationship between education, marketing, and law from the perspective of the cost or benefit to the individual involved. Educational approaches, or

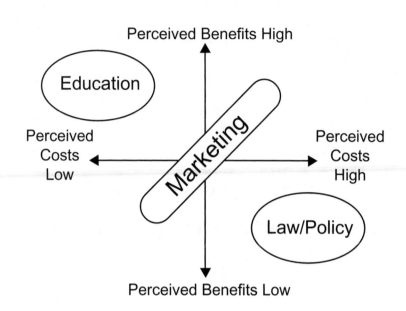

FIGURE 5.1—RELATIONSHIP BETWEEN EDUCATION, MARKETING, AND POLICY/LAW AND THE PERCEIVED COSTS AND BENEFITS TO INDIVIDUALS

Source: Reference 1

simply providing information for decision-making as discussed in chapter 4, might be most appropriate when the benefits of a change in an opinion, attitude, or behavior are obvious and involve minimal cost (effort) to individuals. The "Back to Sleep" campaign of the National Institute of Child Health and Human Development used a direct, informational approach to inform parents that putting babies to sleep on their backs instead of their stomachs cut the risk of sudden Infant Death Syndrome (SIDS).[2] This was a relatively easy behavior for parents to adopt with an extremely high pay-off in terms of peace of mind.

At the opposite end of the spectrum, when the behavior or opinion appears difficult or "costly" to individuals involved and the benefits are not direct, then regulations, policies, or laws might be necessary. Examples include legal controls on advertising and distributing cigarettes, mandatory immunization laws for school entry, and child motor vehicle restraint laws. While the law is concerned with the use of coercion to achieve behavior in a non-voluntary manner,[1] laws tend to act in a persuasive manner, as individuals clearly can choose to disobey many laws according to their personal set of costs and benefits. Just short of laws are community regulations or organizational policies that act on structural factors that might expand or limit personal choices. Sidewalks, noise abatement, flexible workplace hours, or stairwell maintenance are examples of policies or regulations that impact individual health behavior.

Marketing and social marketing efforts fall in the middle ground, and are based on an exchange between a presenter and a consumer. Social marketing can be defined as the design, implementation, and control of programs aimed at increasing the acceptability of a social idea, practice or product in one or more groups of target adopters. The process actively involves the target population, who voluntarily exchange their time and attention for help in meeting their health needs as they perceive them.[3]

Marketing is sometimes confused with the selling or advertising of products, when in fact, these visible (and sometimes annoying) activities occur near the end of the true marketing process. Much time and effort are spent developing a product or service so that it meets the needs of its intended users, with adjustments made to the price, convenience, size, distribution scheme, or other product features. The overall goal is to increase the value and decrease the cost to the intended users. Concepts such as customer satisfaction and "one size does not fit all" derived from for-profit marketing are also key concepts in social marketing, with attention paid to developing programs tailored to the needs of specific groups of users.

Many commercial marketers can become wealthy satisfying the needs or wants of very small groups of users. Social marketing programs for public health often need to consider people as part of larger groups, with the purpose of improving societal health rather than making a profit. Examples of a marketing approach include providing coupons to purchase bicycle helmets at low cost,[4] employer-sponsored programs to provide access to public transportation at reduced or lower cost to discourage driving to work (i.e., to increase walking), and working with bars near college campuses to eliminate low-price drink specials to reduce the volume of student drinking.

Advocacy refers to trying to persuade policy makers to enact regulations, policies, or laws that can potentially impact a large number of people. Such activities can result in large-scale improvement in the health of individuals and can be more efficient and effective than trying to persuade individuals to make behavioral changes one-at-a-time.[5] Medicare reimbursement for adult immunizations, school immunization laws and regulations, and safety belt laws are just a few of many examples of issue advocacy directed towards policy makers that resulted in broad improvements in the health of many individuals in the population. Not surprisingly, policy changes are difficult to achieve as they often encounter political opposition. Detailed discussion of advocacy theories and approaches is beyond the scope of this book; media advocacy is discussed in chapter 6 and communicating with policy makers is covered in chapter 7.

There is synergy between the three approaches of education, marketing, and law. For example, an employer may provide free access to an exercise facility for a limited time period; after the financial incentive ends, self-motivation may increase for some individuals and they may continue to exercise regularly. And, while there are significant penalties for young drivers caught drinking and driving, many drivers are not aware of the laws. Education to increase awareness of the laws, the penalties, and the peer disapproval that can result from being caught can increase the intended effects that simply creating laws alone cannot achieve.[6]

Trying to persuade individuals to make positive health-related changes by using messages to increase their self-motivation is the most common type of persuasive communication used in public health. This is the focus of the remainder of the chapter.

OVERVIEW OF PERSUASIVE HEALTH COMMUNICATION APPROACHES AND THEORIES

Many persuasive approaches and theories have been used over the past 50 years to encourage individuals to make behavioral changes from disciplines as diverse as communication, psychology, sociology, political science, education, and public health. An extensive review of these literatures is beyond the scope of this chapter; instead, a limited number of theories most commonly used in persuasive health communication are discussed.[7]

Many early public health education efforts were based on the assumption that providing information would create knowledge that reliably led to a change in attitude, and that change would subsequently lead to behavior change. Decades of research have demonstrated that while knowledge, attitude, and behavior are, indeed, related, the interaction is not direct and involves other mediating factors.

One model and four theories have reached particular prominence in the practice of health communication. They are often used individually or in some combination to predict behavioral responses to persuasive communication. They include the Precede-Proceed Model,[8] Social Cognitive Theory (originally called Social Learning Theory,)[9] Theory of Reasoned Action,[10] Stages-of-Change Theory (also referred to as the Transtheoretical model),[11] and Diffusion of Innovations Theory.[12]

The Precede-Proceed Model provides an overarching view of the many factors associated with any health behavior change and is based on a community health promotion framework (Figure 5.2).[8] It is particularly useful for examining structural and social obstacles to behavior change, while the remaining theories pertain more to individual-level psychological constructs.

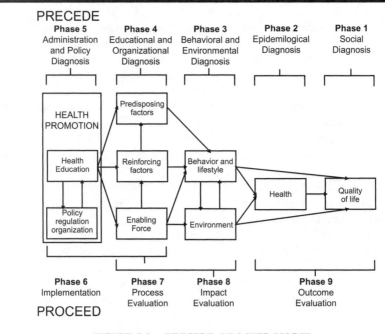

FIGURE 5.2—PRECEDE–PROCEED MODEL

Source: Reference 8

Precede-Proceed includes a needs assessment phase that examines the "*predisposing, reinforcing,* and *enabling constructs in educational/environmental diagnosis and evaluation (Precede)*", and an implementation phase consisting of "*policy, regulatory,* and *organizational constructs in educational and environmental development (Proceed)*". This model has formed the basis for many public health initiatives in the United States over the past 20 years. The model emphasizes the role of predisposing, enabling, and reinforcing factors that influence individual or group health decisions. Predisposing factors include existing beliefs, attitudes, and values (e.g., cultural or ethical norms) that influence whether a person will adopt a behavior. Enabling factors are largely structural, such as the availability of resources, time, or skills to perform a behavior. Reinforcing factors include family and community approval or discouragement that influence behavioral change sustainability

The Precede-Proceed Model is especially valuable for examining a communication effort within a larger context. It often becomes evident that other people and factors outside the individual need to be considered in communication efforts. Prior to committing to a skill-based behavior such as quitting smoking, an individual may need to acquire another skill such as effectively negotiating a behavior change with someone else (e.g., with a spouse who smokes and who is not ready to quit). High neighborhood crime rates may need to be reduced before individuals adopt a walking exercise regime. Often, individual change and group communication strategies may need to be tried simultaneously or sequentially to be effective.

Individual behavior change theories from psychology are at the forefront of health promotion efforts in the United States and elsewhere for areas such as HIV prevention, weight loss, smoking, dietary change, and substance abuse rehabilitation.[7] In essence, Social Cognitive Theory and the Theory of Reasoned Action provide the psychological reasons for the "why, what, and how" for communications designed to promote behavior change, while the Stages-of-Change model provides the "who and when" used for audience segmentation and sequencing interventions.

In Social Cognitive Theory, human behavior is considered the result of a constant interaction between the person and their environment.[9] A key feature of this theory is that individuals must have confidence in their ability to perform a specific behavior, which is referred to self-efficacy.[9] Self-efficacy is based on knowledge and skills (behavioral capability), expectations for the outcome of performing the behavior, value placed on achieving these expectations (expectancies), and reinforcement for performing the behavior. Individuals may either develop self-efficacy for behavior by mastering a series of simpler steps or by observing others perform the behavior and experience the outcome (i.e., observational learning or modeling).

The modeling aspect of Social Cognitive Theory is commonly applied to persuasive health communication. It is based on the belief that people can learn about, rehearse, and master a new behavior by observing role models (often within a dramatic context), then evaluating for themselves whether the modeled behavior is desirable or not. It has been used in many public health situations, ranging from youth tobacco use to domestic abuse prevention programs.[7] Weight-reduction programs often feature a peer-like or a celebrity spokesperson who has successfully lost weight using the product or program being advertised.

The Theory of Reasoned Action,[10] developed in 1980, was "intended to explain virtually all behaviors over which people have the ability to exert self-control,"[13] by predicting individual behavior by expressed intentions. This theory differentiates the expectations from Social Cognitive Theory into groups: one pertaining to expectations about a person's own beliefs and the relative benefits of the behavior, and the other to a person's perceived social norms (e.g., beliefs about how friends and family members feel about the new behavior). The Theory of Planned Behavior[14] adds a third dimension to behavioral intention: perceived behavioral control, or the extent to which an individual believes they are at liberty to perform a behavior.[15] The Theory of Planned Behavior also relates to the Precede-Proceed Model, as it can be used to help explain how predisposing factors are formed within an individual, and how reinforcement works.

Public health messages developed using the Theory of Reasoned Action or Theory of Planned Behavior are persuasive to the extent that they positively influence beliefs about behavior or perceived social norms. This model has been used in mammography screening programs, hypertension control ("Do it for yourself and the loved ones in your life"), youth tobacco prevention (positioning tobacco use as unpopular among social groups), sexually transmitted disease prevention programs, and other interventions.[7] Its popularity, in part, is due to the ease with which behavioral intentions can be solicited for program evaluation. The third individual behavior change model is Stages-of-Change.[11] The basic premise of this model is that health behavior change is a process, not an event. Individuals are likely to make changes when behavior change assets (facilitating factors) outweigh barriers to change (hindering factors). The goal of a public health intervention is to identify and reduce barriers to change and enhance behavior change assets.

Stages-of-Change refers to the five cognitive-behavioral stages that individuals move through when adopting and maintaining a new behavior (Table 5.1). In the precontemplation stage (1), people are not currently considering changing their behavior either because they are unaware of a need to change, they have not considered changing it, or they do not want to change it. In the contemplation stage (2), people are considering a behavior change but have not committed to doing so. In the preparation stage (3), people are actively planning to change their behavior in the near future. The action stage (4) occurs when people have begun to make the change to the new behavior in the short term (usually less than 6 months), and it is followed by the maintenance stage (5), successful adoption of the new behavior for a period of time (usually for 6 or more months). Box 5.1 is an example of persuasive communication based on Stages-of-Change theory.

BOX 5.1

To help address the problem of HIV infection, intervention efforts (based on knowledge gathered from research studies) were launched in several local communities with high risk populations.[16] Public health professionals designed a communication intervention based on Stages-of-Change model.[11] The goal of the project was to move people towards adopting HIV prevention behaviors: avoiding high risk sexual practices and IV drug use.

Communication activities were designed to persuade persons who were already contemplating making a change to prepare to make a change; those who were preparing to make changes to take action, and to encourage those who had made changes to maintain them. Messages featured stories and pictures of role models from within the communities who had successfully made changes; stories were printed in a variety of formats and distributed by community volunteers.

**TABLE 5.1—APPLYING STAGES-OF-CHANGE MODEL TO
PERSUASIVE COMMUNICATION PLANNING**

Stage	Definition	Potential Communication Messages
Precontemplation	Individuals are unaware of problem, have not thought about change, do not want to change	Increase awareness, personalize risks and benefits
Contemplation	Individuals are thinking about a change in near future	Encourage and motivate people to make specific plans
Preparation	Individuals have made a plan to change	Help create a concrete plan of action and set short-term goals
Action	Implementing a specific plan to change	Assist with feedback, problem solving, social support, and reinforcement
Maintenance	Continuing the desired behavior or repeating a periodic action(s)	Assist in coping, provide reminders, find alternatives, handling relapses

Source: Reference 11

There are two aspects that make this theory so appealing for persuasive public health communication First, message content and delivery can be tailored and targeted towards people who are in each of the different stages. For example, a physician counseling a pregnant woman to quit smoking might inform her about dangers to the baby if she is in precontemplation; discuss how to gain family support and reduce barriers to cessation such as alternative stress reduction methods if she is in preparation; or note in her chart the need to provide supportive suggestions at each prenatal visit if she has begun to quit. Second, stages can be scored from one to five, thus providing outcome data that can be used for program evaluation is readily available, e.g., by measuring the number of people who moved from one stage to another. Thus, the Stages-of-Change Theory provides a practical approach for segmenting target audiences for communication planning.

There is one well-established community-based (population) theory that the public health practitioner may use to begin influencing collective thinking. Diffusion of Innovations[12] describes how new ideas, practices, or products spread throughout a population. The diffusion process refers to the innovation itself, the process used to communicate the innovation, and the characteristics of the system or environment in which the process occurs (context).[17,18] It has been used to successfully model diffusion in many fields other than public health.[12]

In Diffusion of Innovations, population groups are characterized by the speed at which they adopt an innovation such as a new idea, product, or behavior. The six groups, which roughly follow a bell-shaped curve, are innovators, early adopters, early majority adopters, late majority adopters, and laggards.[12] The most common use of this theory in health communication is to use messages that attempt to raise awareness among early adopters; this is because persons in this group are often opinion leaders who can influence others to adopt the innovation. Innovators (the initial group to adopt a new idea, practice, or product) are rarely targeted by marketers because they are usually seen as "too different" from the majority of the population, they usually represent a relatively small group, and they are more likely to change without prompting.

Motivational approaches may be most appropriate for majority adopters, while a more effective approach for late adopters may focus on barriers preventing use of the innovation.[17,18] For example, when cholesterol screening was first introduced as a prevention strategy for cardiovascular disease, mass media campaigns suggesting "know your number" were first targeted to health care professionals and opinion leaders in high visibility spots, such as in airports, and through professional journals. A next wave of promotional efforts carried this message to a broader public that was more receptive from the word-of-mouth information transmitted by the opinion leaders and physicians.

PURPOSE AND AUDIENCE

The ideal outcome of persuasion-oriented communication is that persons exposed to the message will adopt the recommended behavior. Realistically, this is difficult to achieve on a population-wide basis because most behaviors are complex. Most people are unwilling to change existing health behaviors without compelling reasons to do so or unless barriers are reduced. Thus, behavior change campaigns often must be multi-faceted, designed to reduce barriers and increase incentives within the environment and to motivate individuals to change.

With a more limited scope and capacity, most persuasive communication efforts focus on increments of change, such as helping people address the key concepts that are reliable predictors of behavior change (for example, perceptions of personal vulnerability, belief in the efficacy of the recommended practice, and belief in their ability to implement the recommended practice). Thus, the specific purposes for persuasive communication are to change awareness (knowledge), beliefs, attitudes, values, readiness, skills, self-efficacy, or self-esteem.

The public health practitioner's purpose and approach to persuasive communication in the general population will vary from situation to situation. Box 5.2 illustrates the importance of creating a persuasive message with a realistic and modest purpose. The message does not describe the types of screening tests, data on colorectal cancer, or frequency of screening. Instead, the communication purpose is to raise awareness that individuals can do something to reduce their risk of colorectal cancer and to encourage people to take a specific action—discuss screening with their doctor at their next visit.

BOX 5.2

A well-liked leader in a medium-sized community recently died of colon cancer at the age of 53. A public health practitioner in the local health district decides to use this as an opportunity to encourage all adults aged 50 and older to receive routine colorectal cancer screening. She works with members of the local chapter of the cancer society to discuss how to increase colorectal cancer screening. They determine that a simple message from a well-known citizen carried in a widely distributed brochure and multiple media interviews will reach adults over age 50 and fit their small budget.

The practitioner directs the design of an inexpensive and visually attractive brochure. Using a positive tone, the simple message encourages adults who are 50 or older to discuss colorectal cancer screening with their doctor at their next appointment. The brochure is distributed by the local cancer society to flu shot clinics, local health care providers' offices, churches, libraries, and senior centers. The practitioner also enlists the help of a 50-year old retired professional athlete well known in the community to help in the effort. She contacts local television and newspaper health reporters about the colorectal cancer screening campaign and the involvement of the ex-athlete. News stories carrying the message from the athlete to "discuss colorectal cancer screening with your doctor at your next visit" receive widespread publicity in the community.

Understanding the audience is essential to effect persuasive communication with the general public. As with efforts to inform the general public, audience segmentation, literacy, numeracy, culture, language, and preferred communication channels all need to be considered prior to developing a persuasive message. As mentioned in the previous chapter, secondary and sometimes tertiary audiences are often used in persuasive efforts targeted towards the general public.

Because communication is an exchange process between message senders and receivers, it cannot be assumed that an audience will value information simply because it is important from a public health perspective. Rather, it is necessary to find out how the audience sees an issue from their perspective. For example, middle-aged adults may be motivated to improve their nutrition and exercise habits to reduce their risk for chronic disease because they have begun to experience body and health changes and understand their vulnerability. Young adults may see the risk of chronic disease as too remote, but may be motivated to improve their diet and physical activity patterns because of the promise of having a higher level of energy.[19]

After deciding on the purpose for the communication and learning the characteristics of the target audience, it is then necessary to assess the level of readiness of that audience to make the desired change and the factors that will facilitate the change or construct barriers. Communication objectives, which are intermediate steps, can then be set which are specific, attainable, prioritized, measurable, and timely.

Objectives can be based on one of the models described earlier in the chapter. For example, the Stages-of-Change Theory could be used to create objectives based on awareness, stimulating contemplation, encouraging a trial, or seeking repeated performance of the behavior; Social Cognitive Theory could be used to set objectives for creating self-efficacy for performing a behavior or to model a behavior and its outcomes.

MESSAGE DEVELOPMENT, MEDIA AND CHANNEL SELECTION, AND EVALUATION

Developing the content of messages was introduced in chapter 2. Content depends on the purpose and the audience, i.e. what is the target audience supposed to do after receiving the message?

Messages cannot persuade people, however, if they are not attended to. Therefore, a critical component of message development is that messages must be presented in such a way that they attract attention and convey personal relevancy to the audience. In the field of health communication this is referred to as message framing. Framing is necessary because the general public is exposed to a multitude of messages that compete for their attention, and they usually have more immediate needs that take precedence over public health issues.

Message framing begins with identifying the appeal of the proposed action in the eyes of the target audience, followed by supporting statements that add to the value of the benefits and minimize the barriers. The only way to do this effectively is to pretest messages with members of the intended audience (chapters 2 and 4). Programs to promote youth smoking prevention, for example, have found that a message promoting nonsmoking as the norm for youth (such as, adolescents will fit in better with their peers if they don't smoke) is more effective than messages stressing the threat of dying from lung cancer. Although poor health and early death are important supporting arguments, the cost of cigarettes, smelly hair and clothes can be raised and reinforced in messages to teens.

In addition to content, message framing also includes tone, format (appearance), spokesperson (or voice), and source. Tone refers to the emotional level and overall style of the communication. The tone and format of messages need to be tailored to targeted audiences. When people see or hear a communication, they almost instantaneously (and unconsciously) filter out messages that do not seem relevant based solely on presentation style and appeal.

This tendency to rapidly assess and "tune out" messages is why message design is so important. For example, messages that resemble a music video may be "invisible" to parents but carefully observed by their children. And, messages delivered by "someone like me" are almost always favored over messages delivered by authority figures or celebrities. Finally, messages sponsored by a recognized public health or medical source are usually perceived as more credible than those sponsored by a commercial source.[20]

A final issue about framing is the use of emotion or affect in persuasive communication. Negative affect (or "fear appeals") can be highly effective for engaging the attention of some audiences.[21] It can also be used to heighten motivation and precipitate action, but only when the recommended behavior is easy to adopt.[22] Positive affect has been shown to gain audience attention, heighten motivation, and precipitate action. In contrast to negative affect, it may have the additional advantage of minimizing "defensive avoidance," such that people shun the message when the recommended behavior is difficult to adopt.[23] This aspect of positive affect can be readily observed in consumer advertising, such as the use of a positive tone for smoking cessation aids, weight loss products, and exercise devices.

The channels through which messages are delivered to audiences are closely related to message content. Decisions about message delivery warrant careful consideration, and such decisions are influenced by several factors: channels preferred by audiences, likelihood of multiple message exposures, and affordability and access for practitioners. Although mass media channels such as television and radio can reach a large number of people, production and advertising costs can be prohibitive, and attention gained by news coverage is usually fleeting. This suggests that practitioners seek out other channels in addition to mass media. Depending upon the target audience and topic, public health practitioners may prefer to create partnerships with others such as health care providers, voluntary health organizations, public institutions, religious institutions, and employers to deliver messages to the public. Communication channels for delivering persuasive messages to general public audiences are the same as for informational messages covered in chapter 4.

A relatively new development in developing persuasive communication is the use of information technology (the Internet) to develop and produce for an "audience of one." Most of the aforementioned theories and communication variables are actualized in "tailoring," where information is collected from a participant and fed into a computer program that generates some form of material based on their readiness to change a behavior and other personal characteristics, including cultural or ethnic identity.[24] The term "tailoring" itself has come to take on this meaning of using interactive technology to develop a custom-fit communication product. Earlier uses of the term have been re-defined as "targeted" (meaning communications are directed to a group sharing common characteristics).

Evaluation of communication messages is essential to understanding whether they were effective (chapter 2).[20] There are many examples in which supposedly persuasive communication efforts take on a life of their own but are never examined as to whether they actually have had a positive impact. Evaluation should be viewed as tool for improving communication efforts, not as a threat. It needs to be included in the campaign as part of the advance planning, not as an afterthought. Admittedly, outcome evaluation is difficult, especially if resources and people are limited, but some effort to assess exposure to messages through process evaluation is almost always feasible (e.g., number of meetings and attendance, number of news stories).

Planning, conducting, and evaluating persuasive communication for the general public has been studied extensively. Readers are referred to references 20, 25, 26, and 27 for a more thorough discussion of these topics.

SUMMARY

The strategies for persuading a public audience to adopt new behaviors include education, marketing, and law, policy, or regulation. Numerous behavior change theories and their associated methods cluster around this core spectrum, all based on a premise of increasing the value of a behavior and reducing its costs. The Precede-Proceed Model stresses the influence of outside factors such as resources and community norms. Social Cognitive Theory, the Theory of Reasoned Action, and Stages-of-Change Theory all stress the role of individual-level factors leading to behavior change. Diffusion of Innovation is a community-level theory used to describe the process by which new innovations are adopted by population groups.

Because persuading people to make changes is difficult, most communication efforts focus on the antecedents of changes such as changing awareness (knowledge), beliefs, attitudes, values, readiness, skills, self-efficacy, or self-esteem. A thorough understanding of the audience including demographics, literacy, numeracy and their readiness for change is important for developing persuasive messages. Developing communication objectives, framing messages to get the attention of audiences, pretesting, communication channel selection, and evaluation are the final steps.

Understanding how general public audiences can be persuaded to adopt healthier behaviors will remain a major challenge for practitioners. Practitioners will need to cooperate with persons familiar with effective persuasion techniques, as too many health professionals still operate under the belief that merely providing information to increase knowledge will result in behavior change.

CHAPTER 5 ENDNOTES

1. Rothschild ML. Carrots, sticks and promises: a conceptual framework for the behavior management of public health and social issues. *J Marketing* 1999;63:24-37.
2. American Academy of Pediatrics and Selected Agencies of the Federal Government. Infant sleep position and sudden infant death syndrome (SIDS) in the United States [joint commentary]. *Pediatrics* 1994;93:820.
3. Lefebvre RC, Flora JA. Social marketing and public health intervention. *Health Educ Q* 1988;15:299-315.
4. Abularrage JJ, DeLuca AJ, Abularrage CJ. Effect of education and legislation on bicycle helmet use in a multiracial population. *Arch Pediatr Adolesc Med* 1997;151:41-44.
5. Brownson RC. Epidemiology and health policy. In: Brownson RC, Petitti DB, eds. *Applied Epidemiology: Theory to Practice.* New York: Oxford University Press; 1998; 349-387.
6. National Institute on Alcohol and Alcoholism. *How to Reduce High- Risk College Drinking: Use Proven*

Strategies, Fill Research Gaps. Final Report of the Panel on Prevention and Treatment. Bethesda MD: National Advisory Council. Task Force On College Drinking, National Institute on Alcohol and Alcoholism, National Institutes of Health; April 2002. Available at: http:www.collegedrinking prevention.gov/Reports/ . Date accessed: June 10, 2002

7. Glanz K, Lewis FM, Rimer BK, eds. *Health Behavior and Health Education: Theory, Research, and Practice.* 2nd ed. San Francisco: Jossey-Bass; 1997.

8. Green LW, Kreuter MW, Deeds SG, Partridge KB. *Health Education Planning: A Diagnostic Approach.* Mountain View, CA: Mayfield; 1980.

9. Bandura A. *Social Learning Theory.* Englewood Cliffs (NJ): Prentice Hall, 1977.

10. Ajzen I, Fishbein, M. *Understanding Attitudes and Predicting Social Behavior.* Englewood Cliffs; NJ: Prentice-Hall; 1980.

11. Prochaska JO, DiClemente CC. Stages and process of self-change of smoking: towards an integrative model of change. *J Consult Clin Psychol* 1983;51:390-395.

12. Rogers EM. *Diffusion of Innovations.* 4th ed. New York: The Free Press; 1995.

13. Institute of Medicine. *Health and Behavior: The Interplay of Biological, Behavioral and Societal Influences.* Washington, DC: National Academy Press; 2001.

14. Azjen I, Madden TJ. Prediction of goal-directed behavior: attitudes, intentions, and perceived behavioral control. *J Experiment Social Psychol* 1986;22:453-474.

15. Alcalay R, Bell RA. *Promoting Nutrition and Physical Activity through Social Marketing: Current Practices and Recommendations.* Sacramento, CA: California Department of Health Services; 2000.

16. O'Reilly KR, Higgins DL. AIDS community demonstration projects for HIV prevention among hard-to-reach groups. *Public Health Rep* 1991;106:714-720.

17. Green LW, Gottlieb NH, Parcel GS. Diffusion theory extended and applied. In: Ward WB, Lewis FM, eds. *Advances in Health Education and Promotion: A Research Annual.* Philadelphia (PA): Kingsley; 1991, pp. 91-117.

18. Oldenburg B, Hardcastle DM, Kok G. Diffusion of Innovations. In: Glanz K, Lewis FM, Rimer BK, editors. *Health Behavior and Health Education: Theory, Research, and Practice.* 2nd ed. San Francisco: Jossey-Bass; 1997:270-286.

19. Parvanta CF, Freimuth V. Health communication at the Centers for Disease Control and Prevention. *Am J Health Behav* 2000;24:18-25.

20. Rimer BK, Glanz K, Rasband G. Searching for evidence about health education and health behavior interventions. *Health EducBehav.* 2001;28:231-248.

21. Reeves B, Newhagen J, Maibach EW, Basil M, Kurz K. Negative and positive television messages: Effects of message type and memory context on attention and memory. *Am Behavioral Scientist* 1991;34:679-694.

22. Pfau M. Designing messages for behavior inoculation. In: Maibach EW, Parrott RL, eds. *Designing Health Messages.* Newbury Park (CA): Sage; 1995:99-113.

23. Monahan JC. Thinking Positively: Using positive affect when designing health messages. In: Maibach EW, Parrott RL, editors. *Designing Health Messages.* Newbury Park, CA: Sage, 1995, p. 81-98.

24. Kreuter MW, Farrell D, Olevitch L, Brennan L. *Tailoring Health Messages: Customizing Communication Using Computer Technology.* Mahwah, NJ: Lawrence Erlbaum Associates, 1999.

25. Academy for Educational Development. *A Tool Box for Building Health Communication Capacity.* Washington, DC: Academy for Educational Development; 1995. Contract No. DPE-5984-Z-00-9018-00. Sponsored by the United States Agency for International Development.

26. Andreasen AR. *Cheap but Good Marketing Research.* Homewood, IL: Business One-Irwin; 1988.

27. Andreasen AR. *Marketing Social Change: Changing Behavior to Promote Health, Social Development and the Environment.* San Francisco: Jossey-Bass; 1995.

SUGGESTED READINGS AND RESOURCES

Alcalay R, Bell RA. *Promoting Nutrition and Physical Activity through Social Marketing: Current Practices and Recommendations.* Sacramento, CA: California Department of Health Services; 2000.

Glanz K, Lewis FM, Rimer BK, eds. *Health Behavior and Health Education: Theory, Research, and Practice.* 2nd ed. San Francisco: Jossey-Bass; 1997.

Kreuter MW, Farrell D, Olevitch L, Brennan L. *Tailoring Health Messages: Customizing Communication Using Computer Technology.* Mahwah, NJ: Lawrence Erlbaum Associates; 1999.

Maibach EW, Parrott RL, eds. *Designing Health Messages.* Newbury Park, CA: Sage; 1995.

Rothschild ML. Carrots, sticks and promises: a conceptual framework for the behavior management of public health and social issues. *J Marketing* 1999;63:24-37.

U.S. Department of Health and Human Services. *Making Health Communication Programs Work: A Planner's Guide.* Bethesda, MD: U.S. Department of Health and Human Services, National Institutes of Health, National Cancer Institute; 1992. NIH publication 92-1493. Available at: http://oc.nci.nih.gov/services/hcpw/home.htm last referenced: February 21, 2002.

Chapter Six

COMMUNICATING PUBLIC HEALTH INFORMATION TO THE NEWS MEDIA

Mike Greenwell, BA

E ffectively using the news media to help improve public health has long been an important component of good public health practice. A practitioner would, quite literally, have to be completely out of touch to not see the overwhelming evidence of the power of the media in Western culture. The power of this influence can be seen, however, as both a curse and a blessing in today's increasingly-cluttered information environment. But it is possible to better understand the news media; by doing so, practitioners will be able to reach both the general public and public policy makers. The purpose of this chapter is to suggest how health practitioners can effectively interact with the news media to further public health goals.

BACKGROUND

The news media is complex and difficult to understand fully, but its potential influence for improving public health is enormous. Although considered in this chapter as a separate audience, the news media is, by definition, a medium or channel, that is, a way to reach other audiences. For public health practitioners, the news media can reach two critically important audiences: the general public and policy makers such as elected officials and administrators.

The news media has changed dramatically since the early 20th century, when it literally meant just newspapers. At the turn of the 20th century, most cities had many newspapers, each catering to the needs of its particular audience, and providing essentially the only source of news. Today, newspaper readership is down dramatically among certain age groups,[1] and some of the largest metropolitan areas have only one newspaper. Television and the Internet are increasingly becoming more important sources for news than are newspapers, especially among persons under 50 years of age.[1] Many local cable television companies and satellite systems provide more than 100 channel choices, and the Internet allows users instant access to news in all corners of the world and the ability for them to access millions of news-oriented web sites.

The news media is part of what is generally referred to as the mass media. The mass media consists of those institutions, both print and electronic, that communicate with large numbers of people who are united by a common focus or interest.[2] Much of the mass media is devoted to entertaining audiences. In contrast, the news media attempts to focus on reporting factual information that is likely to be of interest to general public audiences. Table 6.1 lists the major forms of news media for public health purposes.[3] Television can reach the largest and most heterogeneous audiences; radio, print media (newspapers and magazines), and the Internet tend to reach more specialized public audiences. Public health information from the news media can be communicated to audiences in many ways, including news broadcasts, health programs, editorials, articles, and letters.

The news media is a key audience for public health practitioners for two reasons: the size of the audience it can reach, and its essential role in influencing what people think about (agenda setting).

There are an estimated 100 million households in the United States watching television several hours every day,[4] and tens of millions of Americans listen to the radio or read a newspaper daily. Thus, despite declining audience shares, a health story on a national network news program or in a major daily newspaper can reach hundreds of thousands or in some cases, millions of persons. For example, an article in *USA Today* is estimated to reach 28% of adult Americans.[1] During the height of the anthrax crisis in 2001, a television news package prepared by CDC was rebroadcast 923 times and had an estimated audience of 50.2 million in a two day period.[5] But it is not only the general public who are exposed and influenced; elected officials and public administrators also pay attention to information covered by the news media.[3]

In addition to reaching large audiences, the news media has long played a critical role in determining what events, issues, or people are considered newsworthy. This is referred to as agenda setting.[3] In 1922, Walter Lippman wrote that the "mass media are like the beam of

TABLE 6.1—TYPES OF NEWS MEDIA AND MEANS OF COMMUNICATING PUBLIC HEALTH INFORMATION

Medium	Means of Communicating
Television	News broadcasts, news programs, health programs, talk shows, editorials, paid advertising, public service announcements
Radio	News broadcasts, news programs, health programs, editorials, talk shows, paid advertising, public service announcements
Newspapers (print)	Feature stories (e.g., front page); health or lifestyle section stories; editorials; op-ed articles; letters to the editor; sports, business, or arts stories; paid advertising
Magazines (print)	Feature stories; health or lifestyle section stories; editorials; letters to the editor; sports, business, or arts stories; cartoons; paid advertising
Web Sites	Feature stories; health or lifestyle stories; sports, business, or arts stories; paid advertising

Source: Adapted from Reference 3

a searchlight that moves restlessly about, bringing one episode and then another out of darkness into vision;"[6] in 1963, Bernard Cohen said that "the press may not be successful much of the time in telling people what to think, but it is stunningly successful much of the time in telling people what to think about."[7]

Because of the size of the audiences and the frequency with which people are exposed to the media, its influence is pervasive. Striking evidence of the power of mass media was provided in 1982 when actor Rock Hudson died from AIDS; and again in 1991, when basketball star Magic Johnson announced that he had been infected with HIV. After the announcement of Rock Hudson's death, the number of news media calls to the Centers for Disease Control and Prevention's (CDC) Office of Public Affairs increased from a few thousand per year to more than twenty thousand per year in a short period of time. After Magic Johnson's announcement at a national press conference, the CDC AIDS hotline was overwhelmed with calls, receiving 120,000 call attempts in one 24-hour period.[8] During the anthrax crisis in 2001, a CDC hotline that had not been widely promoted received 18,000 calls from the public over a three month period, while the CDC website had over 21 million visits.

Not only does the news media reach large audiences and help set the agenda for what people think or talk about, it is also an important source for health information. Few issues rival health for its ability to garner public interest and attention; only interest in political figures and events in Washington, D.C. or international affairs begin to compare—and then usually only during times of crisis or scandal.[9]

In a national survey of adults, television was reported as the number one source for health information (39%),[9] ranking higher than health professionals (37%). Respondents reported that the news media influenced their own behavior: 35% reporting that they had talked with their doctor about a medical condition as a direct result of seeing a story about it in the media, and 54% reporting that they changed a health behavior (e.g., diet) because of something reported by the media.

The most common interaction between public health practitioners and the news media involves working with news reporters, either through interviews or press conferences. The remainder of this chapter focuses on understanding how the news media works and communicating with reporters to help further public health goals.

PURPOSE, AUDIENCE, AND MESSAGE

Prior to communicating with news media representatives it is vital to consider purpose, audience, message, message delivery, and timing.

Whether communication is reactive or proactive is the first consideration. If a news reporter contacts a public health practitioner, he or she is obviously already interested in some aspect of a public health story, so access is not a problem. For most reactive communication activities, reporters will view practitioners as an appropriate and reliable source for obtaining data or some other form of public health information. Proactive communication, or getting the news media to take interest in a public health topic or issue, is much more difficult. Framing messages to gain media access requires creation of messages that are considered newsworthy.

Whether reactive or proactive, it is still necessary to decide the purpose of the communication activity. Is the goal to simply inform or to persuade individuals to change behavior, or to advocate for a policy? Closely related to the purpose is the audience to be reached through the news media; is it a broad public audience, a specific segment of the general population, or elected officials? Audience segmentation (chapters 2 and 4) influences decisions to be made about interactions with the news media.

The message, or the "what" of public health communication, is the next consideration. In other words, what's the point? Questions such as, "What action would we like the audience to take?" and "What are we asking the audience to do with this information?" are critical to designing the content and format of the health messages that will be delivered. It may be found that the information to be released is not ready, or that it has too many unanswered questions to be presented publicly.

The single overriding health communication objective (SOHCO) is the core of the message, and ideally should be what would appear in the lead paragraph of a newspaper article or in a television, radio, or Internet news report. (The SOHCO is discussed in more detail later in this chapter.)

MESSAGE PRODUCTION, DELIVERY, AND TIMING

Message production and delivery are very important for proactive media communication. If information is being released for a segment of the population who does not read newspapers—younger audiences[9]—there is no need to ask the print media to cover the story.

Timing is also a consideration. For reactive communication, it is essential to respond to requests as soon as possible, especially from newspaper reporters, as they usually have short deadlines of, at most, a few hours. The situation is variable among reporters from other media, but a rapid response to requests is still important. Even if a story is not scheduled to appear for a few weeks, practitioners will have additional time to decide whether to respond to a request, assess potential audiences, and develop SOHCOs.

Timing is also important for proactive communication. Some public health topics such as fireworks injuries or drinking and driving, have a seasonal or holiday "peg" that can gain media attention.[3,10] Anniversaries of well-known events or providing additional information when a topic is already in the news (for instance, when a celebrity is diagnosed with a preventable injury or preventable type of cancer) increase the likelihood of media interest.[3] Conversely, getting media interest in a health-related topic is very difficult if there is a concurrent story receiving heavy coverage such as a political scandal or severe weather conditions.

GENERAL CHARACTERISTICS AND RECOMMENDATIONS FOR COMMUNICATING WITH THE NEWS MEDIA

There are many different situations for communicating public health information with news media representatives, as well as nuances for each specific medium. Nevertheless, there are some overriding characteristics of the news media and general recommendations that can help guide communication efforts with these audiences.

CONSIDER THE BUSINESS ASPECTS OF NEWS MEDIA AND THE COMPETITION FOR STORIES

Fundamentally, the news media is big business. A part of the changing mass media landscape over the past two decades has been the merger of media institutions and the consolidation of news media outlets.[11] The news media reflects the free enterprise system in which it operates, and is subject to the same forces as any other business. As such, the news media is dependent on its audience interest in being consumers of its products to stay in business. Or, as A. J. Liebling said in 1961, "The function of the press in society is to inform, but its role is to make money."[12] The fact that mass media is a business inevitably raises the issue of the influence of advertising revenues on the type of stories that are covered. Several studies have found that magazines that accept tobacco advertisements are less likely to carry stories about the health effects of tobacco use;[13] further studies have shown this to be especially true in women's magazines.[14,15]

Although health-related stories are commonly covered by the news media,[16] there is much competition as to which stories will be covered. This is most evident for television, where the amount of time devoted to news is limited, but is also true for other news media outlets. The implications of this competition are important: if practitioners want the media to cover a public health issue, it must be deemed newsworthy, and framing for access is necessary.[3] By contrast, if the communication is reactive because a reporter has contacted a practitioner, this represents an opportunity to reach a large audience and the communication activity needs to be an important priority.

Understand the Culture Clash Between Science and News Media

News reporters and scientists have divergent approaches and goals that can lead to conflict.[16] Table 6.2, although it contrasts mass media (rather than just news media) priorities with those of public health, is illustrative of the potential conflicts. News reporters seek information that is definitive, timely, and interesting or relevant to intended audiences, and they are trained to seek answers from multiple points of view. In contrast, science (including the science behind public health practice) uses a much different approach. Science is based on hypothesis testing, a long term perspective, uncertainty, and the very real possibility that current beliefs and recommendations often change based on new evidence. It should also be acknowledged that with the exception of highly-trained health or science writers, most news media reporters are not "mathematically inclined" and may have trouble with numeracy.[17]

As a result of this conflict, news media stories commonly overstate views. For example,

TABLE 6.2—CONTRAST BETWEEN MASS MEDIA AND PUBLIC HEALTH GOALS

Mass Media Goals	Public Health Goals
Entertain, inform, or persuade	Educate
Make a profit	Improve health of the public
Reflect society	Change society
Address personal concerns	Address societal concerns
Focus on short term events	Focus on long term outcomes
Present two or more points of view	Discount or dismiss unsubstantiated claims
Deliver salient pieces of information	Create understanding of complex information
Provide definitive (certain) answers	Acknowledge uncertainty and realize that conclusions can change

Source: Adapted from Reference 16

it has been said that prominently featured health stories stress one of two things: new hope or no hope. Thus it is not surprising that promising research of a particular drug's effect on cancer cells was heralded as a "cure for a cancer"[18] despite the fact that the research was done solely with laboratory mice. Perhaps the fundamental conflict between scientists and reporters has been summarized best by Brooke Gladstone: "science is about questions and that journalism is about answers; science is for the ages while journalism is for the moment."[19]

RECOGNIZE NEWSWORTHINESS

What is news? Although it may often seem like a mystery as to why news media focus on some issues over others, there are a number of factors that determine whether a reporter considers a topic or issue to be newsworthy (Table 6.3).[3,20] Failure to recognize these factors can lead to unnecessary and often counterproductive, proactive communication efforts, such as issuing inappropriate press releases.

News, by definition, must be something that is new. With the exception of infectious disease outbreaks, natural disasters, or acute environmental or occupational exposures, most public health issues are not new, so developing different angles or approaches for presenting information (reframing) is important.[3,10,21] A good example of using a new approach occurred with tobacco control efforts during the 1980s and 1990s, with the emphasis shifted away from the health effects of smoking on smokers themselves, and greater emphasis placed on "unfairness" of health effects among nonsmokers exposed to environmental tobacco smoke and on advertising that targeted children and teenagers.[21]

News is information that the audience needs, that is, it must be relevant to them. Public health practitioners must take an objective look at which information they possess is actually news. A useful paradigm is to imagine how some piece of information would be portrayed to one's neighbors so that the information had meaning for their lives. This may best be summed up by considering what is often the first question a reporter will ask of a scientist reporting findings: "What did you find and what does it mean for our readers?" News is also timely and perishable. The release of information that has recently been covered extensively by the news media greatly diminishes the news value of a story unless it can be portrayed with a new twist or a new context.

TABLE 6.3—CHARACTERISTICS WHICH DETERMINE NEWSWORTHINESS OF PUBLIC HEALTH INFORMATION

New
Relevant to the audience
Timely and perishable
Controversy or conflict
Proximity
Consequence or breakthrough
Human interest or personal angle
Prominence or celebrity
Irony or unusualness
Anniversary or seasonal peg

Source: Adapted from References 3 and 16

News is often about controversy or conflict. In such situations, opposing views will be sought and different sides of a story will be explored. Although conflict or controversy can seem frightening to practitioners, it can result in an opportunity to deliver an important health message that would have been lost had it not been for the controversy. Reporters, for example, may ask the question "were you surprised by the findings?", providing a potential opportunity for practitioners to highlight one or two key points.

Proximity, especially geographic nearness, is another important aspect of newsworthiness. Stories are usually more interesting to audiences if they are based locally. Consequence or breakthrough, that is, events that change or threaten people's lives, also predict the newsworthiness of a story. For example, what is the magnitude of a health problem or will a new approach change how a health problem is addressed?

Presenting a human face ("real people") increases newsworthiness, as stories can be developed around one or more person's experiences. This personal angle can often be used to evoke an emotional response among audiences. Prominence or celebrity, that is involvement of well-known persons such as movie stars or sports figures, can increase interest. This can occur, for example, when a celebrity either develops a health problem or becomes an advocate for a particular activity, program, or policy. Finally, stories that have irony, are unusual, or are linked to an anniversary or seasonal "peg" can sometimes increase newsworthiness.

UNDERSTAND THE PERCEIVED CREDIBILITY OF PUBLIC HEALTH ORGANIZATIONS AND PUBLIC HEALTH PROFESSIONALS AMONG THE NEWS MEDIA

In general, public health institutions have strong credibility among news media professionals. In a 1995 survey, more than 87% of journalists considered persons in academic institutions, professional journals, or government officials to be very or somewhat credible sources of information.[22] By comparison, business organizations and activist groups have much less credibility.

The credibility of persons who present information to news reporters is a function of where they work, as they are perceived as spokespersons for their employer. Because most government agencies, universities, and voluntary organizations have high credibility, practitioners working in these settings will also be considered to be credible. Thus, the most important resource public health officials can offer to those working in the news media is to be a source of unbiased expertise. What this means is that most interviews of public health practitioners by news reporters are done to gather information from expert, unbiased sources, not to generate controversy or conflict.

DEVELOP AND CULTIVATE ONGOING RELATIONSHIPS WITH NEWS REPORTERS

Developing strong and ongoing relationships with news media representatives represents an important, and often neglected, strategy for public health communication. This is even more true at the state and local levels, where reporters are commonly searching for local information for health-related stories (especially newspaper reporters). Building relationships with reporters can be done by promptly responding to requests for information (availability), by translating information into language that can reach the news media audience, and by demonstrating integrity at all times. Being responsive to requests by reporters can result in increased interaction with the media and result in increased receptiveness by media representatives to proactive communication efforts.

RECOGNIZE DIFFERENCES AMONG TELEVISION, RADIO, PRINT, AND INTERNET NEWS MEDIA

Although the characteristics and recommendations in this section apply to all forms of news media, each medium has its own unique characteristics. Television is a highly visual medium that necessitates the use of pictures and usually reaches a broad general public audience. For example, if a story is about the need for children to be more physically active, one approach would be to videotape children at a school where officials have made a strong commitment to have students participate in physical education classes.

Radio audiences tend to be highly specialized based on demographics and preferred interests (e.g., age group, music or talk radio format). This requires a good understanding of audience profiles; for example, targeting stories about drunk driving to radio stations with younger audiences. News stories should be told in a way that is very short and succinct to fit the radio format.

The length and formats of newspaper and magazine articles, and the audiences to be reached, are highly variable, and the writing of the stories is at the discretion of the reporter. Newspaper reporters usually work on short deadlines, so rapidly responding to interview requests or more information is essential. Magazine writers generally write more in-depth articles and deadlines are usually longer.

There has been a great increase in the number of Internet news sites. Most media outlets such as newspapers have their own Web sites, but there are also an increasing number of sites that are only on the Internet.[23,24] These Web sites and the reporters who work for them should be viewed as similar to newspapers and magazines, with the major difference being that stories can be presented to Internet audiences immediately.

CONSIDER APPROPRIATENESS OF COMMUNICATING TO NEWS MEDIA REPRESENTATIVES

Prior to communicating with the news media it is necessary to reconsider the purpose of the communication. Is it appropriate to attempt to interest the media (proactive communication)— is there something newsworthy to report? For reactive communication, consider whether it is appropriate to respond to a news reporter's request for an interview. In reactive circumstances, responding is almost always appropriate, even if to say that there is no new information.

If a decision is made to communicate with the news media, it is essential to let appropriate higher-level staff know about the activity. Managers or administrators may then help decide who should be the appropriate spokesperson to represent the organization or if someone outside the organization (e.g., a member of a voluntary health organization) should do the interview. There are circumstances when practitioners or their managers may decide to refuse an interview; participating in a debate on the merits of proposed state legislation on motorcycle helmets on a talk radio program, for example.

CONTACT AND UTILIZE PERSONS EXPERIENCED IN COMMUNICATING WITH THE MEDIA

Few public health practitioners have time to become experts in the field of media relations, but many public health organizations have some kind of media relations or public affairs staff to provide assistance. It is their job to know the needs and demands of the news media, and to develop professional and proactive relationships with those in the news media business. Media relations or public affairs staff can save much time by relaying basic information, such as deadlines, who else is being interviewed, and recent coverage on the particular subject. At a minimum, practitioners should notify the public affairs staff in the organization when news media requests are received, as they can help in preparations for the interview.

If a public health practitioner does not have access to public affairs or communications staff in their organization, the best approach in handling media interviews is to seek advice from persons in other organizations such as state or federal public health agencies, or to contact a local university with a school of journalism.

Although much of the chapter focuses on proactive communication with the news media, being able to effectively respond when the news media is covering a real or perceived public health crisis is equally important. Trying to hide from the media in a time of crisis is never a good strategy. Tips on handling media crisis situations are discussed in the Barriers and Challenges section later in this chapter.

SPECIFIC RECOMMENDATIONS FOR COMMUNICATING WITH THE NEWS MEDIA

Whether the communication is proactive or reactive, there are some specific recommendations that can improve interaction with news media representatives.

PREPARE FOR THE INTERVIEW

A public health official being asked to participate in an interview with the press may be either so intimidated by, or impressed with, the potential impact of the news media that he or she may feel somewhat at the mercy of the reporter. It may be practical to view this relationship as more "give and take," and understand that both groups need each other and must acknowledge each other's needs.

Perhaps most important, public health practitioners do not have to agree to do an interview immediately just because a reporter is on the other end of the phone line. The practitioner should take some time to prepare by learning about the context of the interview. For example, after learning the context, practitioners can agree to call back later in the day and use this time to review notes, summarize information, and create a SOHCO.

There are a few simple questions that the person to be interviewed, or the public affairs or public information staff need to ask, including the deadline, whether the interview is live or taped, the subject of the story, others being interviewed, and controversies (Table 6.4).

Practitioners are under no obligation to respond to questions for which the answer is not known, and should refer reporters to more knowledgeable persons if questions cover topics for which they are not prepared to answer. If follow-up information is promised to a reporter, it should be provided as promptly as possible.

TABLE 6.4—QUESTIONS TO ASK NEWS REPORTERS PRIOR TO AN INTERVIEW

What is the deadline for completing the interview?
Is the interview to be taped or live?
What exactly is the story about?
Who else has been interviewed?
What are some of the controversies being explored?

DEVELOP A SOHCO AND USE IT

The most important thing to do before a media interview is to develop the single over-riding health communication objective, or SOHCO. The SOHCO must be the most important thing that is said to a reporter; it would ideally appear in the lead paragraph of a story in the newspaper or in the first sentence or two of a radio, television, or Internet news broadcast. An effective SOHCO usually consists of one sentence that sums up the most important aspect of what is being communicated, followed by several statements that support or qualify that sentence.

The SOHCO is essential to make certain that the key message is provided but it must be brief and concise to meet the confines of news media reports. A good SOHCO has a clear intent and a strong "take home" message. Table 6.5 provides examples of SOHCOs that have been used at CDC in recent years.[25-29] Always remember that when providing health information designed to stimulate change, the audience usually has the choice of

TABLE 6.5—EXAMPLES OF SINGLE OVERRIDING HEALTH COMMUNICATION OBJECTIVES (SOHCOS) USED BY THE CENTERS FOR DISEASE CONTROL AND PREVENTION

Utilization of Preventive Services, Behavior Risk Factor Surveillance System–United States, 1995[25]	Use of four preventive services–flu shot, pneumococcal pneumonia vaccine, mammography, Pap smear–among the elderly falls short of national goals in many states. These findings suggest that simply having health insurance does not ensure that these important preventive services will be used and changes in service delivery and programs tailored to the needs of older adults may be needed.
Incidence of Initiation of Cigarette Smoking–United States, 1965-1996[26]	A new study released today by the Centers for Disease Control and Prevention found that each day an alarming number of young people join the ranks of regular smokers. The study estimated that 1.2 million young people under the age of 18 became daily smokers in 1996–more than 3,300 young people every day.
Fatal Occupational Injuries—United States, 1980—1997[27]	Despite the decline of both the number and rate of traumatic occupational fatalities, an average of 16 fatalities still occur each day. The National Institute for Occupational Safety and Health acknowledges that significant improvements in occupational health and safety have been made, but also recognizes that occupational injuries and fatalities continue to be a major public health concern.
Vitamin A Deficiency Among Children—Federated States of Micronesia, 2000[28]	Vitamin A deficiency is a severe public health problem among pre-school children in the Federated States of Micronesia. This problem very likely extends to other segments of the population and needs a comprehensive long-term national strategy to promote sustained improvement in vitamin A status.
Hepatitis B Outbreak in a State Correctional Facility, 2000[29]	Hepatitis B vaccination of inmates would prevent ongoing hepatitis B virus transmission in correctional facilities, as well as infection in inmates after release into the community.

Sources: References 25-29

doing something else. Marketers have long acknowledged the competition in designing advertising campaigns and provided clear and simple messages; public health practitioners can use lessons learned from the marketing world.

The SOHCO should be written and be immediately available during the interview, and it should be stated often during the course of the interview. Figure 6.1 is a planning sheet used for developing SOHCOs at CDC for Morbidity and Mortality (MMWR) articles that can easily be adapted for other situations.

Office of Communication/Media Relations
MMWR FACT SHEET
Single Overriding Health Communication Objective (SOHCO)

In one paragraph, please state the key point or objective of your MMWR submission. This statement should reflect what you, the writer, would like to see as the lead paragraph in a newspaper story or in a broadcast news report about your submission.

List three facts or statistics you would like the public to remember as a result of reading or hearing about your article?

What is the main audience or population segment you would like this article to reach?

Primary	Secondary

What is the one message the audience needs to take from this article?

Who in your office will serve as the point-of-contact for media questions?

Name: Degree(s):   Phone:*

Title: Division/Center:

Date and time available:

FIGURE 6.1—OUTLINE FOR DEVELOPING HEALTH COMMUNICATION OBJECTIVE (SOHCO) FOR MMWR ARTICLES

Source: Centers for Disease Control and Prevention

SPEAK IN NON-TECHNICAL LANGUAGE AND USE NUMBERS SPARINGLY

Speaking in language that is quotable will greatly lessen the chance of being misquoted. In other words, speak in the language of everyday conversation as much as possible. For example, scientists may want to avoid clichés because they appear to show a lack of original thinking, but among the general public, people use clichés often because they are widely understood. Technical terms, if used, must be introduced slowly, and they need to be thoroughly explained.[30]

If the story involves numbers, pick a few and stick with them. Most news stories will not accommodate many numbers, so if one or two numbers are essential, mention them to the reporter, or he or she will simply decide which numbers to include. For example, if a condition causes 36,500 deaths per year, it is probably more effective to say "this condition causes the death of 100 Americans each day." Numeric analogies (chapter 3) can be used effectively to make the numbers more real an provide context. Simple visuals such as a pie chart or line graph can help reporters translate numbers for their audience.

ANSWER QUESTIONS APPROPRIATELY

To handle interview questions, it is essential to anticipate what the questions will be and to practice the answers. This normally involves creating a list of questions and answers, or Qs and As. These Qs and As should include not only the obvious questions, but also potentially difficult ones. Anticipating the "nightmare scenario" questions, and practicing answers that address them, can reduce anxiety.

A simple "yes" or "no" is rarely a sufficient answer to an interviewer's question, even during the most hostile of interviews. Answers must be elaborated upon, examples or illustrations can be given to provide clarity, and other views or positions can be acknowledged and explored. It is equally important for a person being interviewed by a reporter to realize that there is no such thing as an "off the record" response. Especially for those working in the public sector, everything that is said, from the moment the interview begins until the reporter hangs up the phone, or the news crew is leaving the parking lot, is on the record.

Knowing that not every question will be one that is welcome, or even appropriate, should not be seen as a lost opportunity. A technique known as bridging allows the person being interviewed to acknowledge the question, say that it is not one that can or should be answered, and return back to the main message planned when developing the SOHCO. Every opportunity to refer to the single-most important communication objective should be utilized. The use of some transition phrases can make this bridging to the SOHCO a little easier such as: (1) What is important to remember is. . . ; (2) What I think you are really asking is. . . ; (3) What I can tell you about our recommendation is. . . (4) What I'd really like to emphasize is. . . ; (5) Let me put this in perspective. . .

During the interview practitioners should not use the words "no comment" when asked questions, as this may imply that information is being hidden. Table 6.6 provides a list of tips for media interviews that can provide helpful insights for improving interviews with news media representatives.

MEDIA ADVOCACY

Most public health communication efforts emphasize using the news media to reach individuals within the general public. However, the media can be a tool for encouraging

TABLE 6.6—TOP 20 TIPS FOR IMPROVING MEDIA INTERVIEWS

1. Know why you are doing the interview
2. Know to whom you are speaking—who is the audience?
3. Coordinate the interview with your public affairs office (if applicable)
4. Establish interview ground rules immediately (subject, location, length) and stick to them
5. Review the facts even if it's in your area of expertise
6. Prepare by anticipating questions and preparing answers—play the devil's advocate
7. Remember that everything you say is "on the record"
8. Establish a friendly, cooperative, but professional atmosphere
9. Relax—you are the expert (many reporters are generalists who rely on you for information)
10. Listen carefully to each question; if necessary, include the question as part of your answer
11. Speak in plain English; avoid scientific jargon and acronyms
12. State the conclusion or single overriding health objective first
13. Use short quotes to help make your main points quickly
14. Avoid making personal commentary or expressing personal opinions
15. If you don't know, say so; if appropriate, offer to follow up with the reporter
16. Gently correct the reporter if he or she has the facts wrong
17. Keep cool—do not argue with reporters or repeat negative statements
18. Never say "no comment"
19. Avoid hypothetical or "what if" questions.
20. Always provide promised material to a reporter in a timely manner

broader social change by attempting to persuade policy makers to adopt or eliminate programs, resources, policies, laws, or regulations (discussed in detail in reference 3.) Media advocacy seeks to influence the selection of topics by the mass media and shape the debate about these topics, and to contribute to the development and implementation of social and policy initiatives that promote health and well-being based on the principles of social justice.[3] Media advocacy is one part of an overall strategy to effect social change.

Media advocacy consists of three key elements: setting the agenda, shaping the debate, and advancing the policy. Setting the agenda consists of trying to draw the attention of the news media to a particular issue and helping them to see it as newsworthy. Since few public health problems are new, this usually involves reframing problems to be newsworthy, often referred to as framing for access.[3,21]

The second step of media advocacy is shaping the debate. This requires overcoming the tendency of the news media to present health problems as individual problems that can readily be overcome by "willpower" or "pulling oneself up by one's bootstraps." Because of the short-term focus and emphasis on individuals, the underlying policies, political decisions, and barriers making it difficult for individuals to act in more healthy ways are rarely explored by the media.

The final step in media advocacy is advancing the policy. The news media will not willingly advance policy goals, no matter how laudable. Instead, advancing the policy means to continue efforts to change policy through multiple means (e.g., legislation, referenda, organizational or public pressure on key policy makers), as well as attempting to keep the media focused on the problem and the "solution" being advocated. To do so requires that the news media be provided with new ways to portray the story in different contexts, and that this be done quickly, given the short-term focus of the media.

An important note of caution about media advocacy: with the exception of editorial writers, news media representatives are quite wary of being considered a part of moving a particular social or policy goal forward. Reporters would readily say that their job is not to influence policy, or even to educate the public on a particular issue. Instead, they believe their job is to inform the public of relevant social issues.

CHALLENGES AND BARRIERS

FAILING TO SEEK NEWS MEDIA ATTENTION

Probably the most important challenge when communicating with the news media is simply not doing so.[21] Many practitioners either do not want to do so, do not view it as part of their responsibility, have multiple competing priorities, or do not know how to communicate with the news media. It can be challenging to work with the media, as information can be taken out of context, conflicts can occur, and the impact is not always immediately evident. But given the influence and importance of the media for reaching both the general public and policy makers, and the interest of the public in health issues, more efforts are needed to communicate with the news media.

DIFFICULTY GETTING NEWS MEDIA ATTENTION FOR MANY PUBLIC HEALTH ISSUES

Unfortunately, because of the reality of the journalistic approach and the media business, some important public health issues receive little media attention, while others receive a great deal of attention. Given these realities, it is not surprising, then, that Ebola virus, which has never killed anyone in the United States, has been the subject of movies and many news reports, while public health issues such as alcohol-related illnesses or occupational diseases receive little media attention.[21] Overcoming these inherent media biases toward short-term and dramatic problems requires much creativity to develop new messages and approaches that are considered newsworthy. Box 6.1 provides an example of how a creative approach was used to get news media attention for trends in adult obesity.

PUBLIC HEALTH CRISES

Communication with the media plays a key role in public health crisis situations. Never was this more evident than during the anthrax attacks in 2001. CDC was thrust into one of the most significant public health crises in history with the incidents of the intentional release of anthrax in several locations in the U.S.[32] The immediate public and media interest in the story resulted in a record number of inquiries, and required the use of crisis com-

---

BOX 6.1

The October 26, 1999 release of a study entitled "The Spread of the Epidemic of Obesity in the United States" in *JAMA*[31] garnered front-page newspaper and national broadcast news coverage. This story described the increase of overweight and obesity in America, but used a slightly different perspective than that used for a study published only a few weeks earlier in the *New England Journal of Medicine*.

The way in which the obesity information from the *JAMA* study was presented to the news media had a major impact on their interest in the story. The adage that "a picture speaks a thousand words" is never so applicable as in garnering news coverage for a particular issue. In the case of public health stories, the adage may be adapted to say "a well-designed map or chart speaks a thousand words."

In the *JAMA* article, all materials prepared by the authors included camera-ready maps that depicted the spreading epidemic of obesity (Figure 6.2); these maps appeared in many of the articles written about the study. An image of an epidemic of a non-infectious disease moving across the U.S. added much interest to a story already covered many times in the press.

munications skills at nearly every level throughout the agency. Crises requiring effective communication with the media, however, occur at the state and local levels during outbreaks of infectious diseases, perceived or actual environmental or occupational exposures, mass psychogenic illness, natural or manmade disasters, or in response to dangerously inaccurate health information from other sources.

It is essential that practitioners in public health agencies communicate with the media in an appropriate and timely manner during these situations. Such communication, when done well, can facilitate communicating specific actions or precautions that individuals should take to avoid or cope with the health problem (e.g., drink bottled water only). If media communication is done poorly in these situations, it can lead to distrust, cynicism, and charges of a "cover-up."

An important part of communicating during a crisis such as bioterrorism is to not over-reassure, and to acknowledge uncertainty when it exists (chapter 13), as leaders are seldom criticized for stating uncertainty.[33] As mentioned by risk communication expert Peter Sandman, "Journalists will often ask whether they are getting told the truth, rarely whether you know the truth."[33] Several general steps are important when communicating with the media in these situations.[34] These include to: (1) stay calm; (2) build an advisory team; (3) designate a team leader; (4) designate a spokesperson; (5) get the facts; (6) be honest; and (7) alert key supporters. It is essential that a consistent message be communicated by a public health agency in these situations.

After the events of September 11, 2001 and the subsequent anthrax attacks, there has been increased interest in developing and refining crisis communication plans for public health and other organizations. There are numerous resources available to help guide practitioners and agencies in the development of crisis communication plans. (Further information on communicating with the media during crisis situations is available in references 33-39.)

Being Too Trusting or Open with News Reporters

The opposite problem of failure to communicate with media representatives is being too trusting or open with reporters. As mentioned before, news is a business and good reporters are adept at asking questions and attempting to develop a trusting relationship with interviewees. However, a practitioner may forget that reporters are always looking for news, and that answers that can provoke controversy or conflict are newsworthy items. It is essential to always remember that everything said to a reporter could potentially appear on the television, radio, newspaper, magazine, or an Internet site the next day.

Being Misquoted or Having Information Taken Out of Context

It is inevitable that the more often a practitioner communicates with reporters, the greater the likelihood of being misquoted or having information taken out of context. If this happens, a decision needs to be made as to whether to respond or not. Misquotes or out of context information should usually be ignored unless they are egregious.

If the reporter badly misstated an important fact that must be corrected, then the reporter should be contacted and advised of the error; the media outlet may or may not print or broadcast a correction or clarification. If the misprint was in a newspaper or magazine, another option is to write a letter-to-the-editor or an op-ed article to clearly address the issue.[40]

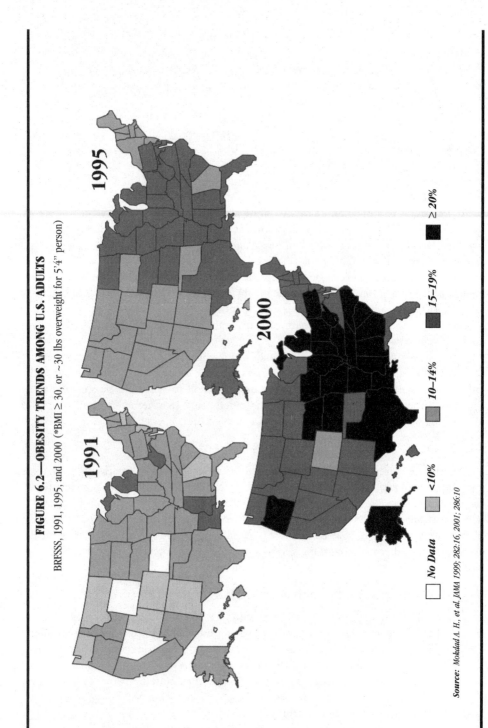

FIGURE 6.2—OBESITY TRENDS AMONG U.S. ADULTS

BRFSS, 1991, 1995, and 2000 (*BMI ≥ 30, or ~30 lbs overweight for 5'4" person)

Source: Mokdad A. H., et al. JAMA 1999; 282:16, 2001; 286:10

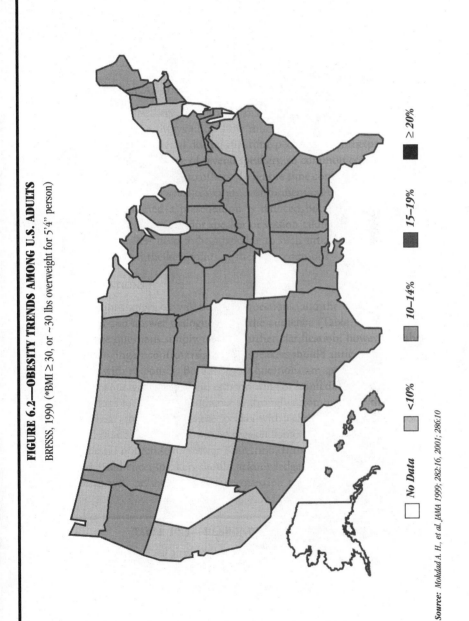

FIGURE 6.2—OBESITY TRENDS AMONG U.S. ADULTS

BRFSS, 1990 (*BMI ≥ 30, or ~30 lbs overweight for 5'4" person)

No Data   <10%   10–14%   15–19%   ≥ 20%

Source: Mokdad A. H., et al, JAMA 1999; 282:16, 2001; 286:10

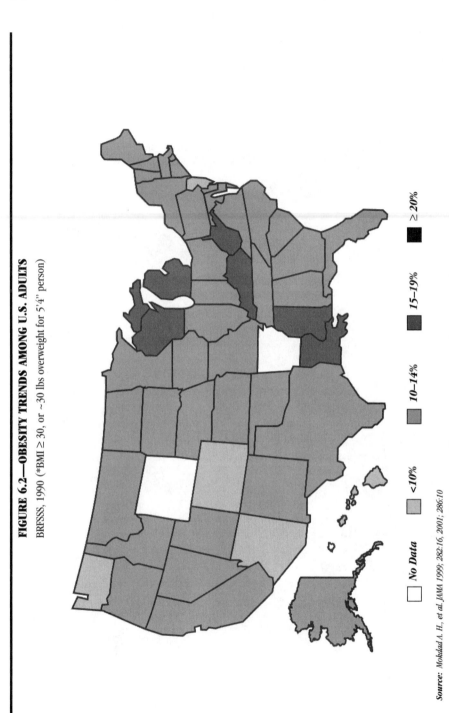

FIGURE 6.2—OBESITY TRENDS AMONG U.S. ADULTS

BRFSS, 1990 (*BMI ≥ 30, or ~30 lbs overweight for 5'4" person)

No Data   <10%   10–14%   15–19%   ≥ 20%

Source: Mokdad A. H., et al, JAMA 1999; 282:16, 2001; 286:10

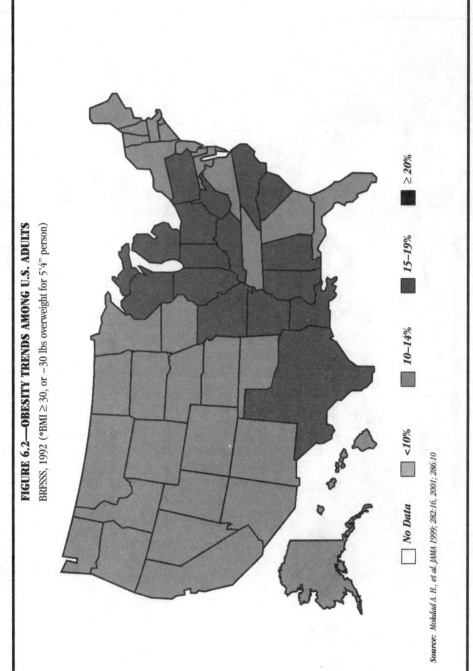

FIGURE 6.2—OBESITY TRENDS AMONG U.S. ADULTS

BRFSS, 1992 (*BMI ≥ 30, or ~30 lbs overweight for 5'4" person)

No Data   <10%   10–14%   15–19%   ≥ 20%

Source: Mokdad A. H., et al. JAMA 1999; 282:16, 2001; 286:10

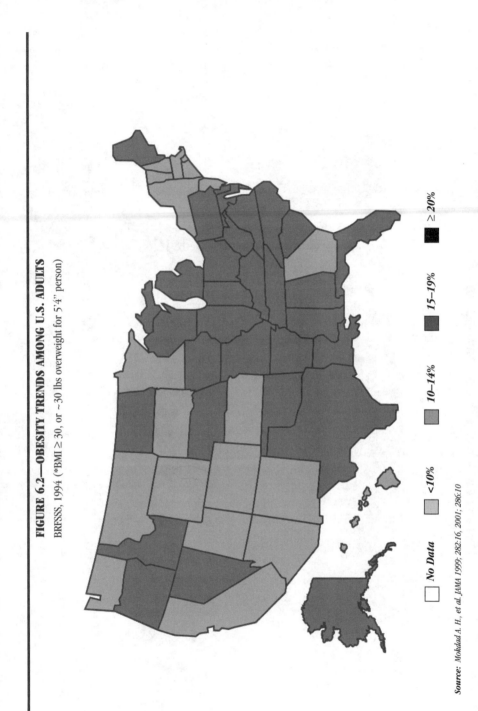

FIGURE 6.2—OBESITY TRENDS AMONG U.S. ADULTS

BRFSS, 1994 (*BMI ≥ 30, or ~30 lbs overweight for 5'4" person)

No Data <10% 10–14% 15–19% ≥ 20%

Source: Mokdad A. H., et al. JAMA 1999; 282:16, 2001; 286:10

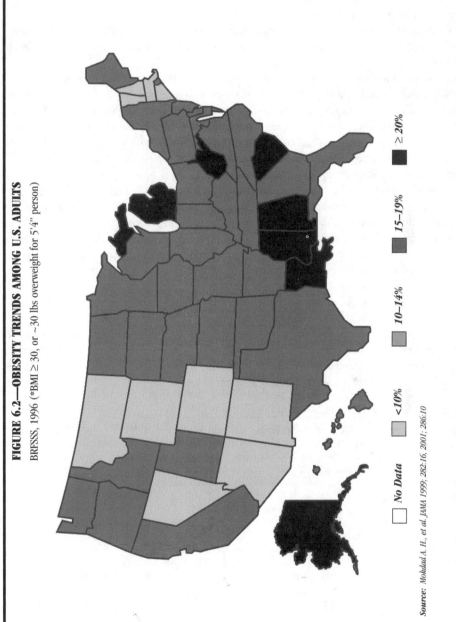

FIGURE 6.2—OBESITY TRENDS AMONG U.S. ADULTS

BRFSS, 1996 (*BMI ≥ 30, or ~30 lbs overweight for 5'4" person)

No Data   <10%   10–14%   15–19%   ≥ 20%

Source: Mokdad A. H., et al. JAMA 1999; 282:16, 2001; 286:10

SUMMARY

The mass media play an important role for public health practice because of their reach and their role in agenda setting. The major forms of mass media for public health are television, radio, newspapers, magazines, and the Internet. Whether communication with news media representatives is reactive or proactive, it is essential that the purpose, audience, message, timing, and communication channel be understood prior to the communication activity.

When communicating with news media representatives, it is necessary to recognize several general media characteristics and considerations. These include the business aspects of news media, understanding the culture clash between science and the news media, recognizing newsworthiness, and knowing that practitioners usually have high credibility as a source for information. Other considerations include developing ongoing relationships with reporters, recognizing the differences among mass media outlets, considering the appropriateness of doing an interview.

Specific recommendations for communicating with the media include utilizing persons experienced in media communications, preparing for the interview, developing a SOHCO, speaking in non-technical language, and answering questions appropriately. Media advocacy is a means for promoting change in social policy through the media, and it involves agenda setting, shaping the debate, and advancing the policy. Challenges and barriers include failing to seek news media attention, difficulty getting media attention for public health issues, crises, being too trusting of reporters, or being misquoted.

The changing face of mass media in last decade of the 20th century presents both a profound dilemma and a great opportunity for public health practitioners. The proliferation of mass media outlets, including the Internet require multiple and often innovative approaches to reach audiences. Understanding and utilizing television and the Internet news media more effectively will be of increasing importance, especially because of the decline in newspaper readership among younger persons.

CHAPTER 6 ENDNOTES

1. The Pew Research Center for the People and the Press. Internet News Takes Off. Available at http://www.people-press.org/med/98rpt.htm. accessed July 12, 2001.
2. Watson J, Hill A. *A Dictionary of Communication and Media Studies.* New York: Arnold; 1995.
3. Wallack L. *Media Advocacy and Public Health.* Newbury Park, CA: Sage; 1993.
4. A.C. Neilsen. Web site address: http://www.acneilsen.com. accessed July 12, 2001.
5. Ogilvy Worldwide. *CDC Anthrax Update.* NY: News Broadcast Network; 2002.
6. Lippmann W. *Public Opinion.* New York: Free Press; 1965.
7. Cohen B. *The Press and Foreign Policy.* Princeton, Princeton University Press; 1963.
8. Jorgensen C, Nunnally B, Dunmire R. *Forging partnerships in public information: state and federal agencies working together in HIV prevention efforts.* Paper presented at: 120th Annual Meeting of the American Public Health Association, November 10, 1992; Washington, DC.
9. Rodale Press. *Survey of Public Opinion Regarding Health News Coverage.* Emmaus, PA: Rodale Press; 1998.
10. Wallack L. *News For a Change: An Advocate's Guide to Working With the Media.* Thousand Oaks, CA: Sage; 1999.
11. Bagdikian B. *The Media Monopoly.* Boston: Beacon; 1987.
12. Liebling AJ. *The Press.* New York: Ballentine; 1961.
13. Warner K. Cigarette advertising and magazine coverage of the hazards of smoking. *N Eng J Med.* 1992;326:305-309.

14. Gerlach K. Cancer coverage in women's magazines: What information are women receiving? *J Cancer Educ.* 1997;12:240-244.
15. Hoffman-Goetz L. Cancer coverage and tobacco advertising in African-American women's popular magazines. *J Community Health.* 1997;22:261-270.
16. Atkin C, Wallack L, eds. *Mass Communications and Public Health.* Newbury Park, CA: Sage; 1990.
17. Paulos JA. *Innumeracy: Mathematical Illiteracy and its Consequences.* New York: Vintage Books; 1990.
18. Kolata G. Hope in the lab. A special report: a cautious awe greets drug that eradicates tumors in mice. *New York Times.* May 2, 1998, 1.
19. Gladstone B. Interview on "Morning Edition" with Robert Lee Hotz [transcript]. National Public Radio. June 4, 1998.
20. Meyer P. News media responsiveness to public heath. In: Atkin C, Wallack L, eds. *Mass Communication and Public Health: Complexities and Conflicts.* Newbury Park, CA: Sage; 1990.
21. Siegel M, Doner L. Marketing Public Health: *Strategies to Promote Social Change.* Gaithersburg, MD: Aspen; 1998.
22. Strategic Communications and Research and Duquesne University Bayer School of Natural and Environmental Sciences. *Environmental Journalism Survey.* Denver: Strategic Communications and Research; 1995.
23. WebMD Web site: http://www.webmd.com. accessed July 12 2001
24. HealthScout Web site: http://www.healthscout.com. accessed July 12 2001.
25. Centers for Disease Control and Prevention. Use of clinical preventive services by Medicare beneficiaries aged ≥ 65years—United States, 1995. *MMWR.* 1997;46:1138-1143.
26. Centers for Disease Control and Prevention. Incidence of initiation of cigarette smoking—United States, 1965-1996. *MMWR.* 1998;47:837-40.
27. Centers for Disease Control and Prevention. Fatal occupational injuries—United States, 1980-1997. *MMWR.* 2001;50:317-320.
28. Centers for Disease Control and Prevention. Vitamin A deficiency among children—Federated States of Micronesia, 2000. MMWR 2001;50:509-512.
29. Centers for Disease Control and Prevention. Hepatitis B outbreak in a state correctional facility, 2000. *MMWR.* 2001;50:529-532.
30. Gastel B. *Health Writer's Handbook.* Ames, IA: Iowa State University Press; 1997.
31. Mokdad AH, Serdula MK, Dietz WH, Bowman BA, Marks JS, Koplan JP. The spread of the obesity epidemic in the United States, 1991-1998. *JAMA.* 1999;282:1519-1522.
32. Centers for Disease Control and Prevention. Recognition of illness associated with the intentional release of a biologic agent, October 2001. *MMWR.* 2001;50:893
33. Fox J. *How To Work With The Media.* Newbury Park, CA: Sage; 1993.
34. Sandman PM. Anthrax, bioterrorism, and risk communication: guidelines for action. Available at: http://psandman.com/col/part1.htm. accessed March 5, 2002.
35. Jones C. *Winning with the News Media: A Self-Defense Manual When You're the Story.* Tampa, FL: Video Consultants; 2001.
36. Wade J, Hicks T, eds. *Dealing Effectively With the Media.* Menlo Park, CA: Crisp Publications; 1992.
37. Freeo, SKC. *Crisis Communication Plan: A Blue Print.* Available at: http://www3.niu.edu/newsplace/crisis.html. accessed March 5, 2002.
38. National Education Association. *Crisis Communications Guide and Toolkit.* Washington, DC: National Education Association; 2002. Available at: http://nea.org/crisis. accessed March 5, 2002.
39. Public Relations Society of America. *2002 Crisis Communications Report: Crisis Communications in a Post-September 11th World.* New York City: Public Relations Society of America, Best Practices in Corporate Communications; 2002. Available at: http://www.prsa.org/prc/BestPractices.html. accessed March 5, 2002.
40. National Clearinghouse for Alcohol and Drug Information. *Technical Assistance Bulletin: Working with the Mass Media.* Rockville, MD: Center for Substance Abuse Prevention; 1998.

SUGGESTED READINGS AND RESOURCES

Atkin C, Wallack L, eds. *Mass Communications and Public Health.* Newbury Park, CA: Sage; 1990.

Fox J. *How To Work With The Media*. Newbury Park, CA: Sage; 1993.

Jones C. *Winning with the News Media: A Self-Defense Manual When You're the Story.* Tampa, FL: Video Consultants; 2001.

Siegel M, Doner L. *Marketing Public Health: Strategies to Promote Social Change*. Gaithersburg, MD: Aspen; 1998.

Wallack L, Dorfman L, Jernigan D, Themba M. *Media Advocacy and Public Health*. Newbury Park, CA: Sage; 1993.

Wallack L, Woodruff K, Dorfman L, Diaz I. *News For a Change: An Advocate's Guide to Working With the Media*. Thousand Oaks, CA: Sage; 1999.

Chapter Seven

COMMUNICATING PUBLIC HEALTH
INFORMATION TO POLICY MAKERS

Ross C. Brownson, PhD
Bernard R. Malone, MPA

Policies and the effective allocation of resources can have substantial effects on the health of the public.[1-3] Therefore, health policy makers represent a critical audience for public health practitioners. If information is effectively communicated to policy makers, they will be more likely to develop and implement laws, regulations, and programs that protect and promote the public health. This chapter describes several key methods that are useful when communicating public health information to policy makers.

BACKGROUND

Ideally, policy makers should incorporate scientific information when developing policies, implementing programs, and making management decisions. The use of sound data in supporting a policy initiative is illustrated in the example in Box 7.1.

In reality, however, many decisions are based on short-term demands rather than long-term study, and policies and programs are frequently developed around anecdotal evidence. Existing health data are often under-utilized and sometimes ignored.[6,7] These concerns

---

BOX 7.1

In the field of tobacco control, Oregon enacted Ballot Measure 44 ("An Act to Support the Oregon Health Plan").[4] Despite being outspent by the tobacco industry by 7 to 1, the initiative passed with 56% of the vote. Public health data helped a broad-based coalition to build public support for Measure 44. This information included the health and economic burden of tobacco use, patterns of tobacco use among youth, the prevalence of persons without health insurance, and polling data showing strong public support for a tobacco tax of up to 50 cents per pack. A 1999 report of the Oregon Health Division highlighted the successes to date of the Measure 44 tobacco programming, including the development of 36 county tobacco-free coalitions, 24 school projects reaching 170,000 students, and an 11% decline in per capita cigarette consumption in Oregon since 1996.[5] Advocates also organized a successful lobbying campaign to see that the legislature did not divert tobacco control monies to other uses.[4]

were highlighted over a decade ago when the Institute of Medicine determined that decision-making in public health is often driven by " . . . crises, hot issues, and concerns of organized interest groups."[8]

As described in chapter 1, policy makers include both elected officials such as local or state legislators, and high-level administrators such as heads of departments or agencies, who have the authority to make decisions about laws, regulations, other policies, programs, and resources that can impact many people.

Health policies can be broad in scope, and in addition to laws, may involve organizational practices; therefore, health administrators can have substantial impacts on health policy development and implementation. There is also considerable overlap between the roles and impact of elected officials and administrators. For example, after a state legislature enacts laws and passes budgets, the director of a state health department must decide how resources are to be allocated and where an agency's emphasis should be placed when carrying out various health policies.

Practitioners need to develop a real-world perspective about the role of scientific information in policy making. Even among highly trained individuals in the most favorable settings, it is unrealistic to expect that public health programs will be based solely on what data suggest. Decisions on where public health action should be taken are complex and depend on numerous factors, including preventability, severity, economics, and public interest. Even when public health data are clear and consistent, there are multiple interpretations and numerous policy options.[10] It is also important to remember that, although most scientific discoveries in public health are achieved through incremental advances in knowledge over years or decades, policy makers often want quick and definitive answers to complex questions during crises. Despite these challenges, data from research studies and surveillance systems are the primary tool for practitioners to use when communicating with policy makers, as it is often difficult for people to argue against these "facts."[11]

Although the remainder of this chapter focuses on communicating to policy makers in the public sector, many of the principles and approaches apply equally to communicating public health information to policy makers in private or voluntary health organizations.

CHARACTERISTICS OF POLICY MAKERS

Given the key role and impact that health policies can have on population health status,[3,12] it is essential to understand the general characteristics and factors that apply to key decision-makers in public health settings.

The decision-making process among public health professionals often differs from that in political environments (Table 7.1). In public health and medicine, decisions are often made by one person or by a small number of persons. Conversely, in the political system decisions are often made by consensus.[13] For example, in the U.S. Congress, decisions are made only with the support from a majority of the 435 representatives and 100 senators. There are, however, some important differences between administrators and elected officials, and these are discussed below.

ADMINISTRATORS

In public health agencies and health care organizations, program and agency leaders come from a variety of backgrounds. Often they are talented individuals who have "risen

TABLE 7.1—COMPARISON OF THE PUBLIC HEALTH AND POLITICAL DECISION-MAKING PROCESSES	
Public Health Process: Rational Decision Making	Political Process: Intuitive Decision-Making
Identify problem	Identify problem
Develop options	Place in context
Analyze options	Use judgment
Implement policy	Assess reaction
Evaluate effect	Prepare for next crisis

Adapted from Reference 13

through the ranks" of an agency, yet they may lack formal training in disciplines such as epidemiology or biostatistics. Unlike professions such as medicine or law, no core educational degree is required for professional work in public health. For example, the U.S. public health workforce is estimated at a half million, yet less than half of all employees in public health departments have formal training in public health.[14] In addition, high-level administrators in many public health departments are political appointees who may lack both formal public health training and agency experience.

Thus, administrators may bring a diverse set of skills to the practice of public health; some will be facile with data and statistics, others less so. Because of this, knowing the organizational "culture"—the abilities and preferences of individual administrators, and communication style (e.g., e-mail vs. face-to-face meetings)—is essential in order to effectively present information. Much of this type of knowledge can only be obtained either through direct experience with the individual administrator or through discussions with others who are familiar with his/her background and preferences.

ELECTED OFFICIALS

Governmental policy systems vary widely in their structure and scope.[15] In uni-centric policy systems, such as totalitarian governments, power is concentrated within one governmental authority. Within pluri-centric systems, power is shared by a small number of interdependent actors in government and labor—widespread support of policies is needed for policy implementation, as in Japan and Germany, for example. A multi-centric policy system involves interaction of many autonomous actors, with government serving as the guardian of standards; the democratic system. In this chapter, the descriptions of health policy communication are focused on multi-centric, or democratic, governments.

In a democratic form of government, the role of a legislative body is clearly delineated. Whether at a local, state, or federal level, the purpose of the representative body is to enact rules, laws, or ordinances to be implemented by executive or administrative agents. Many examples of legislative bodies exist in our society, including local city/county councils, state legislatures, and the United States Congress. These bodies have the primary purpose of enacting public policy based on the will of the people in order to direct the executive and administrative units of government charged with responding to society's needs.

Since legislatures are the arena for the formulation of public policy, it is critical to have an understanding of the process whereby legislatures obtain community and citizen input.

Many groups play an active role in the development of the public policy, including constituent groups, activists, citizen groups, advisory boards, and task forces.

When working in the arena of health policies, it is critical to consider the political climate and major societal trends affecting public health and health policies. For example, in the United States, there has been a recent shift regarding the governmental role in health policy from the federal to the state level (devolution)[16]; many believe that innovative programs are more likely to occur at state and local levels rather than at the federal level.

Even when one understands the public health needs and trends, the practice of influencing health policy is as much art as science. Depending on the type of legislative body, numerous opportunities exist to provide formal and informal input into this process. Most legislative bodies divide their focus through the establishment of committees to which members with a particular interest or intent are assigned. Committees are intended to provide an efficient and effective process whereby legislative bills with a common interest or focus can be reviewed, debated, and approved for submission to the larger legislative body. In nearly every legislative body within a large community or state, a specific committee is established for public health issues. In other cases, the committee may focus solely on general health and medical issues under the review of the legislative body, or it may be combined with public welfare or other human service issues.

Whether attempting to work with elected officials or administrators, public health practitioners are too often placed in a reactive mode and may attempt to solve problems under severe time constraints. To be in a position to proactively communicate with policy makers effectively, it is important to establish sound working relationships with elected officials or administrators prior to a crisis. If trust has already been established, policy makers are much more likely to believe public health data and be willing to work with practitioners on a specific issue or problem. Strong relationships are based largely on mutual understanding and respect; once these are established and regularly maintained, practitioners can focus on ensuring that the information they provide to policy makers is of the highest quality. This will reinforce the belief among policy makers that practitioners are experts in a given area.

PURPOSE, AUDIENCE, AND MESSAGE

Practitioners must have a clear understanding of the purpose for communicating, specifically, is the goal to inform or to persuade? There are some instances, especially when practitioners must react to requests of policy makers, in which the communication will be to inform. In these situations, the approach for communicating with policy makers will not differ substantially from the approach used for other audiences.

However, most communication with policy makers is designed to persuade; to obtain support for resources, programs, policies, or regulations. The public health practitioner, then, must take a firm stand on an issue while developing and presenting a clear message based on the scientific evidence. Answering the questions "What is my goal?" and "What message do I want to leave with this individual or group?" as specifically as possible will help avoid interactions that will be vague and unfocused. Note that for governmental employees, persuasive communication efforts directed towards certain policy makers (usually legislators) cannot occur without the permission of a higher-level administrator or an elected executive (e.g., a governor or mayor).

Understanding policy makers, as with any other audience, is crucial. With few exceptions, policy makers are extremely busy and they receive many requests from different individuals and groups asking for support of specific policies or resources. Given this backdrop, the more knowledge that practitioners can develop about policy makers, their operating styles, and the systems in which they work, the greater their chances are for success.

As mentioned earlier, administrators and the organizations they work in vary widely, so consulting with others who are familiar with an administrator is essential. Internet Web sites can be a very useful way to learn about the organization that an administrator manages, and many elected officials have their own Web sites that can provide valuable information about officials—backgrounds, preferences, and voting records. If practitioners will be testifying before a legislative committee, it is likely that some elected officials will be supporters and others will be opponents. Learning about likely proponents and opponents is essential for preparing messages and anticipating counter arguments. The finding and effective use of data from the Internet for a legislative audience is illustrated in Box 7.2.

Regardless of whether practitioners are communicating with administrators or elected officials, these audiences are likely to focus on two general themes: how much it is expected to cost, and who is likely to be adversely affected or otherwise opposed (political considerations).

The message to communicate to policy makers is highly variable and depends on each situation. In brief, the "what" involves deciding on the most concise and important pieces of information that can be used to persuade policy-makers to act. The message should be direct, definitive, and defensible (backed up by the science). If the information or request is to be presented to a legislative committee, it is often helpful to picture one person on the committee to whom one will target the message such as the person who has substantial influence over the committee. It is also necessary to have the opposition in mind and to be prepared to counter their arguments.

Practitioners must anticipate questions about financial resources, such as "How much will this program cost?" or "Will this program save my city or state money?" These issues should be handled carefully, as economic evaluations are complicated. In general, preventive measures taken by public health professionals are not cost saving, but are a good bargain compared with many other well-established practices.[17] Depending on the situation, practitioners may be better off to prepare messages based on expected non-financial benefits to people (improved quality of life for constituents) rather than cost savings.

BOX 7.2

The state public health officer in Missouri was called upon to testify before the Public Health Appropriations Committee regarding plans to expand a program aimed at reducing smoking among pregnant women. The state health department proposed expansion of a limited, pilot program to a program covering one-half of the state's counties. Initial, informal discussions between the health department leadership and appropriations staffers indicated a strong interest in targeting the program toward low income and/or African American women. Because the state collects information on the mother's smoking status on each birth certificate, data were available to help focus the program. Data obtained from the health department's Internet Web site revealed that the highest smoking rates during pregnancy were among low-income women (using Medicaid status as an indicator of income level). Their smoking rate was nearly three times higher than any other population subgroup. This information was key in helping to persuade lawmakers to provide increased resources for this program with a strong focus on smoking cessation among low-income, Medicaid-eligible women.

SELECTING A SPOKESPERSON AND MESSAGE PRODUCTION AND DELIVERY

When communicating with policy makers, who delivers the message, (the spokesperson), can be important. Within an organization, this may mean that a practitioner's immediate supervisor or another person elsewhere in the organization whom the administrator knows and trusts is the best choice.

Sometimes one may be attempting to persuade a single influential elected official. Because of constraints within public health agencies, an "outside" spokesperson may be desirable, such as an articulate health professional with a public health orientation who lives in the official's district. Other potential presenters may include well-known or highly placed individuals from voluntary or private health organizations (chapter 8). Depending on the situation, local, state, or even national celebrities can be called upon to help.

There are several ways to deliver messages to policy makers. These communications may occur in highly structured or less structured settings; the approach and amount of preparation needed depend on the situation and setting. For communicating with administrators, practitioners will likely develop, over time, an understanding of the "corporate culture" and learn from others how certain administrators prefer to receive information. This is especially true in highly-structured organizations that have a distinct "chain of command." Some administrators will prefer e-mail, while others may prefer memos, oral presentations, or telephone interactions.

Communicating with elected officials differs from communicating with administrators. Such interactions can include correspondence, informal meetings, or more formal situations. A hearing, for example, is a highly structured and formal setting for making an oral presentation. In such hearings, a group of elected officials gather in a committee meeting room to hear testimony from experts (witnesses) in the public health field. Witnesses are usually given only a few minutes to make their statements. Therefore, it is critical to be well prepared by have key pieces of information on hand and anticipating responses to counter arguments. Further recommendations for communicating with elected officials are discussed later in this chapter.

GENERAL RECOMMENDATIONS FOR COMMUNICATING WITH POLICY MAKERS

Although there are some important differences between administrators and elected officials, when it comes to communication situations, there are many similarities. The following set of general recommendations can be used for written or oral communication with both audiences, and is intended to complement related descriptions in other chapters.

MAINTAIN THE FOCUS

It is essential to remember and stress the main communication message and stay focused on it. If the nature of one's public health responsibility is to reduce premature death, make that the main message and the focus of the communication. Relate all that is said to that main point—this will underscore the importance of the public health agency's responsibility and will sharpen the attention of the audience to that single message.

GET QUICKLY TO THE POINT

Policy makers are often inundated with requests from others for more resources, new policies, etc. Given this fact, and that communicating with policy makers is usually a proactive act by practitioners, it is essential that the communication activity gets to the main point quickly. Lengthy introductions or background material should be avoided. Early in the discussion, one should state the main message and repeat it often so that the policy maker will develop a clear understanding of the issue and the desired action step. The frequency with which one repeats the key point will be determined by the complexity of the issue and the specific situation.

USE NUMBERS APPROPRIATELY

Unlike other nonscientific audiences, policy makers will generally be more familiar with numbers; they will also be more demanding about the strength and validity of the evidence presented to support a position. Practitioners should always be prepared to explain and defend the scientific basis for their position. This is often accomplished through the use of statistical information. The two most common questions are likely to be: "Which public health statistics should I present?" and "How should this information be presented?" Health indicators (measures of the extent to which program objectives are being reached) can be useful starting places for determining which statistics to present. These indicators are commonly measured and have relevance across population subgroups.[18,19] For example, in developing support for tobacco control legislation, lung cancer mortality rates can be presented at statewide or county-specific levels. It is often useful to risk reduction gains (e.g., lives saved) among various alternatives when several options are on the table.[20] Also, remember that local data works best. An example showing the effective use of data is shown in Figure 7.1; these data were used persuasively to build support for expansion of efforts to control cardiovascular disease in Missouri. Another example of communicating data to policy makers is shown in Figure 7.2; a similar bar chart was used in a U.S. Senate hearing in 1996 to demonstrate the problem of the uninsured over the past several decades.[21]

AVOID JARGON AND CLICHÉS

Excessive use of jargon and clichés will only confuse an audience and may project an attitude of elitism. Not everyone will understand technical terms, and using them runs the risk of losing the support of one or more elected officials who might be potential allies and advocates for one's position. Do not use words that are in vogue, such as "infrastructure" or "modality," as they are overused and sometimes appear to reflect an overly academic or bureaucratic style. The goal is to express, not impress the intended audience.

BE CONCISE

Concise presentations, including summaries of data, are more challenging to prepare than tomes. Practitioners are unlikely to have more than a few minutes to spend with policy makers, therefore the message needs to be short, crisp, and readily understood. If the communication is solely in writing (correspondence or e-mail), a good rule of thumb is that it should be limited to one page with the key points bulleted.

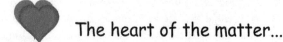

The heart of the matter...

This is the second of three fact sheets designed to highlight the burden of cardiovascular disease (CVD) in Missouri.

Trends and Disparities

 Death from stroke for Missouri women of all races/ethnicity increased during the past four years, reversing a 25-year downward trend.

 Serious cardiovascular health disparities exist for minorities in Missouri. African Americans are 1.4 times more likely to die from CVD than whites.

In 1997, about half of African American women in Missouri were overweight. If the current trend continues, almost all African American women could be overweight by 2010. Being overweight or obese increases one s chance of developing and dying from coronary heart disease and stroke.

The statewide CVD death rate is 195.9 per 100,000. There are stark differences among the counties. The range extends from a low of 148.5 in Howard County to 327.5 inPemiscot County.

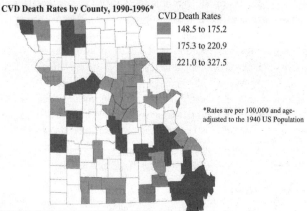

CVD Death Rates by County, 1990-1996*

CVD Death Rates

- 148.5 to 175.2
- 175.3 to 220.9
- 221.0 to 327.5

*Rates are per 100,000 and age-adjusted to the 1940 US Population

Source: MDOH Center for Health, Information, Management and Evaluation

*The Missouri Department of Health has established a statewide Cardiovascular Health Advisory(CVH) Board whose first task was to create*The Missouri Cardiovascular Health State Plan, 2000-2010. *The Plan seeks to raise awareness of CVD as the primary killer of*Missourians *and to coordinate efforts of statewide partners.Look for the Plan to be released in March 2000.*

--*Missouri CVH Advisory Board*

Missouri Department of Health. Division of Chronic Disease Prevention and Health Promotion. Bureau of Chronic Disease Control
(573) 522-2860

FIGURE 7.1—MISSOURI CARDIOVASCULAR DISEASE FACT

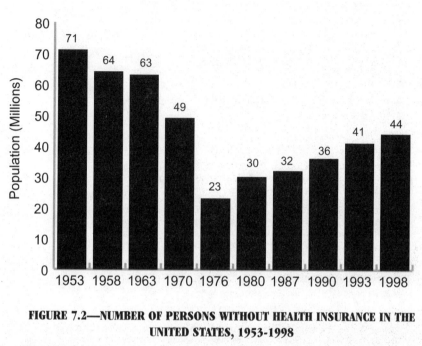

FIGURE 7.2—NUMBER OF PERSONS WITHOUT HEALTH INSURANCE IN THE UNITED STATES, 1953-1998

Adapted from Reference 21

If the communication is a formal oral presentation, a short written summary should also be provided. A one-page handout for the administrator or legislator that summarizes key points is a useful adjunct to the oral presentation (Figure 7.3). A "one-pager" is also a good idea when communicating with policy makers in less structured situations such as individual meetings, as they can help avoid digressions.

BE SPECIFIC AND USE REAL WORLD EXAMPLES

Always use words that clearly state the intent and do not lend themselves to generalization or misinterpretation. A personal example of the need or impact of the program being discussed can have a large effect on the audience and help accentuate public heath data findings. For example, if one was seeking to implement a policy to reduce youth purchase of tobacco, adolescents' testimony on how easy it was to purchase tobacco can be more effective than simply discussing the number of youth who take up smoking.

ADDITIONAL RECOMMENDATIONS FOR COMMUNICATING WITH ELECTED OFFICIALS

The opportunities to impact the debate on public health issues are numerous and diverse. Influence can be direct and one-on-one through personal contact with an individual's elected official, through private or voluntary health organizations, or through other groups such as coalitions.

DIABETES PROGRAM
APPROPRIATIONS

ASTDHPPHE

Association of
State & Territorial
Directors of Health
Promotion and Public
Health Education

FACT SHEET

The Centers for Disease Control and Prevention's Diabetes Program is presently funded at $49.3 million. **The FY2000 Administration budget proposes no funding increase for this program.**

We support a FY2000 appropriation of $100 million. The increase will enable all states to expand their efforts and have comprehensive programs. This year, CDC will provide minimal support ($200,000 avg.) to 34 States for core diabetes control programs, and greater support ($800,000 avg.) to at least 16 States for comprehensive programs.

Basic Facts About Diabetes

- Approximately 15.7 million Americans have diabetes.
- About 2,200 new cases are diagnosed each day in our Nation.
- The American Diabetes Assn. estimates that this disease costs the nation $98 billion a year in medical care, lost wages, and disability.
- Diabetes is the leading cause of blindness among working -age adults. If people with diabetes receive appropriate screening and care, diabetes-related blindness could be prevented in 15,600 individuals a year (65% reduction), resulting in federal government annual savings of at least $470 million.
- Diabetes is the leading cause of kidney failure, affecting almost 28,000 new individuals each year. Diabetes related kidney failure could be reduced by 50%, preventing roughly 14,000 cases and saving over $350 million in dialysis and treatment costs over a 10-year period.
- More than 1/2 of lower-limb amputations occur among people with diabetes - 67,000 diabetes-related amputations are performed annually. With appropriate assessment and patient education, 40,200 diabetes-related amputations could be prevented each year - a 60% reduction, resulting in a savings of over $285 million annually.

CDC's Diabetes Program

CDC supports state and territorial diabetes control programs aimed at reducing the complications associated with diabetes. These programs seek to educate people with diabetes and health professionals about the disease and its complications. The programs identify high risk populations, support early detection and treatment of complications, help improve the quality of diabetes care, and enhance access to diabetes care by improving and expanding services.

FIGURE 7.3—FACT SHEET ON NATIONAL DIABETES CONTROL PROGRAM FOR FISCAL YEAR 2000

OVERVIEW OF FACTORS AND APPROACHES

Table 7.2 lists ten factors and approaches that are essential for effective communication with elected officials.

Knowing the legislative process, approach, and timetable are crucial considerations. For example, meeting face-to-face with elected officials can be a good way to share ideas and thoughts on a particular issue. Frequently, elected officials will remember such individual meetings and consider the input that is made during these interactions. However, legislative time constraints may sometimes render this option impractical or ineffective. Consider that most legislative bodies meet for a specified period of time with a very structured calendar—one that allows little flexibility. The lack of flexibility becomes even more defined as the session moves into its final few weeks. Special committee hearings and caucuses are often held at that time and little opportunity is afforded for individual meetings.

More effective strategies are available in the first few weeks of a legislative session. One option is to provide testimony at public hearings; another is to arrange private meetings with key stakeholders from the community, particularly if they are from the legislator's home district. Success in getting the message out to elected officials to influence the legislative process is greatly affected by timing. The best way to learn how to time advocacy efforts is to consult with people familiar with the legislative process and for practitioners to learn about the policy-making process themselves. An elected official is unlikely to want to visit a local health promotion event scheduled at the same time as an important committee meeting or vote.

Professional groups (e.g., voluntary or private health organizations such as the local medical society) and other "stakeholders" can also influence elected officials (chapter 8). In many cases, legislators will seek out such agents and groups and will actively consider their opinions. The greatest impact will be attained through combining the efforts of local constituent representation with stakeholder groups that have a specific interest in a particular measure.[22]

A clear understanding of the issues, the expected beneficiaries and groups that will be harmed, and the opposition and their arguments are necessary ingredients of success. Relationships with elected officials are not developed at one meeting or during one legislative hearing. As with all other audiences, public health practitioners who plan to be involved in the policy arena will need to find out as much as possible about individual legislators, including their opinions and voting records. "Get-acquainted" meetings that occur at times other than the legislative session and periodic briefings or updates help to build good relationships.

Practitioners should maintain their integrity at all times; it is far better to admit to not knowing an answer than to cover up a mistake. Understanding and respecting the role of legislators is important, as most are hard working individuals who must represent a diverse group of citizens with many different opinions.

Practitioners may underestimate and underappreciate the roles of legislative aides or assistants. Such individuals are the gatekeepers for elected officials, and developing and maintaining strong professional relationships with these individuals can greatly influence the policy-making process.

Active listening to elected officials about their positions and their needs is important, as it shows mutual respect and understanding for the challenges that such officials face when

TABLE 7.2—TEN UNDERLYING QUALITATIVE FACTORS AND APPROACHES FOR EFFECTIVELY COMMUNICATING WITH ELECTED OFFICIALS

Develop familiarity with the legislative process	Every legislative body has its own unique structure, calendar and culture. The process has numerous hearings, floor debates, amendments, conference meetings, and other opportunities within which to provide input.
Show knowledge of the issue	Analysis needs to be done which clearly establishes what problem is being addressed and whether there is a legislative solution. It is useful to answer three questions: Who will this help? Who will it hurt? How much will it cost?
Develop knowledge of the opposition	Elected officials will want to be aware of formal and informal opposition to a given proposal. It is critical that proponents know whom these groups or individuals are, the reasons for their opposition, and the strength of opposition.
Develop an established relationship with legislators	Efforts should be undertaken to have knowledge of key members, their constituencies and their prior records on issues relating to yours. It is important to have "get acquainted" meetings at a time convenient to the elected official and not during the actual session of the legislative body. Periodically providing brief program updates or providing information for he/she to use in his/her district is a useful tool to supporting that relationship.
Maintain integrity	It is essential that your integrity be assured in all dealings with elected officials. If an answer to a specific question is not known say so. If a mistake is inadvertently made, immediately acknowledge it and ask for the benefit of the doubt in future encounters.
Respect their role	Elected representatives are generally doing their best to represent the citizens of their district or region. Advocates should understand that rarely does a legislator represent an area that has universally accepted opinions.
Respect the role of their staff	Legislative staff plays critical roles of gatekeeper and opinion shaper. As with the individual elected officials, it is essential to have a professional working relationship with staff members as well.
Show a willingness to listen	Perhaps the most essential product of conversations with elected officials and advocates is the listening regarding the position of the official or his/her other constituents who may be in support or opposition. Active listening is a learned trait and it is essential to success in this arena.
Be forthright in your position	Let the legislative sponsor know of your support or opposition to avoid public disagreement or embarrassment. A private meeting should be held in which you articulate your position and your rationale. These interactions can help to build a greater appreciation and respect for your position.
Maintain a focus on "the long view" and "the big picture"	Think about issues in the big picture rather than issue by issue. While an elected official may not support your position on one issue, it is important to be able to come back to him/her on future occasions. Remember that there will be other issues, and it is never advisable to "burn any bridges."

doing their jobs. Nevertheless, public health advocates should be forthright and honest about their views and not be afraid to articulate their support or opposition to a position and their rationale.

Finally, working with elected officials to change laws, regulations, or resource apportionments that benefit the health of the public is hard, frustrating work. Practitioners will need to maintain a long-term and big-picture view to be successful in such advocacy work. In addition to working with elected officials, working with many populations to garner their support requires a substantial commitment of time and energy to build the necessary trust between public health practitioners and community members.

PUBLIC HEALTH AGENCIES AND LEGISLATIVE BODIES

For an executive agency involved in a legislative debate or in the development of public policy, the only clear commodity is the possession and dissemination of information. Thus, there are several reasons for taking a systematic approach to presenting information. Reliable information that is provided in a meaningful, comprehensive, yet concise manner is extremely influential in the public policy debate. It can often provide essential background support as to why a particular issue has reached the legislative arena. It also provides reason, instead of emotion, and fact, rather than belief and anecdote, to legislative debates. And finally, it will provide clear evidence of the impact of proposed legislative action.

Credibility is the critical component in being effective at working with a legislative body. Executive agencies are most effective when they have earned the respect of legislators and have a reputation for providing information that is accurate, timely and in manner that is free of error. It is noteworthy that in a survey of 38 state health officers across the United States, the area cited as the greatest need was better skills in working with the state legislature.[23] More recent focus group research suggests that similar abilities, such as negotiation skills are key for public health administrators.[24] The information, whether in support or in opposition to a particular proposal, must be presented in a forthright, yet non-confrontational manner.

TIPS FOR FACE-TO-FACE MEETINGS AND ORAL PRESENTATIONS

A face-to-face meeting with elected officials can be a daunting experience, especially for practitioners who have limited experience in this arena. Table 7.3 summarizes the key points to consider when preparing for such meetings or formal presentations. In addition to these points, remember that the news media can be an important secondary audience at legislative hearings. Public health professionals should consider using language that would make good quotations ("sound bytes") and provide copies of written materials to news media representatives.

In addition to content, tone of voice and body language are also powerful communication tools in helping to persuade audiences. A few techniques will help improve the impact and effectiveness of oral presentations:

1. *Shake hands and make eye contact.* When meeting an official, shake hands and greet him or her with eye contact. In a formal oral presentation, attempt to maintain eye contact with the audience. If there is a large audience, address the committee chairperson or other person in charge of the meeting. Presenters should avoid darting their eyes across the room or to written notes.

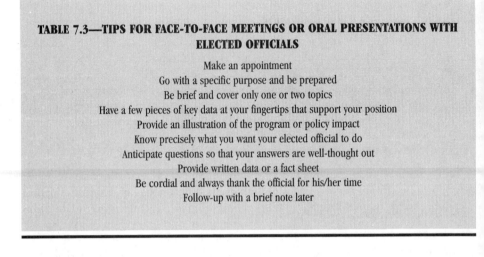

TABLE 7.3—TIPS FOR FACE-TO-FACE MEETINGS OR ORAL PRESENTATIONS WITH ELECTED OFFICIALS

Make an appointment
Go with a specific purpose and be prepared
Be brief and cover only one or two topics
Have a few pieces of key data at your fingertips that support your position
Provide an illustration of the program or policy impact
Know precisely what you want your elected official to do
Anticipate questions so that your answers are well-thought out
Provide written data or a fact sheet
Be cordial and always thank the official for his/her time
Follow-up with a brief note later

2. Sit upright in the chair and appear relaxed and confident. This will convey an appearance of being interested, involved, and assured.

3. Dress appropriately. A practitioner's physical appearance and the manner in which he/she presents the message are clear reinforcements to the message itself. It is generally good practice to dress conservatively (select solid colors over flashy patterns); wear simple jewelry; never wear a hat; avoid shaded or dark glasses unless medically required; and use make-up sparingly. Most importantly, it is essential to look professional so that physical appearance does not detract from the message.

4. Begin with the main message. State the conclusion early and follow up with supporting data and other information.

5. Make the message directly relevant to the elected officials. When facing a rather abstract concept, such as the value of disease prevention, present some concrete examples that illustrate the key point(s). For example, when testifying to the impact of premature mortality from chronic disease in a given city, one might frame the issue in the following way: "Last year, more people died from chronic diseases in this state than live in the city of _____."

CORRESPONDENCE

In addition to the oral presentations, face-to-face meetings, and "one-pagers," correspondence can play a key role when communicating with elected officials. One may communicate in writing to an elected official in three different capacities. As do all citizens, one may express his or her views as a private citizen on a particular public health topic. If corresponding in one's official work-related capacity, permission from a supervisor is often needed to express views on an issue. And finally, one may provide support to a group or coalition and may "ghost write" correspondence on a particular issue.

Table 7.4 provides a list of things to consider when writing letters to elected officials. In addition to these considerations, who signs the letter is also important, especially if more than one individual or organization is represented.

CHALLENGES AND BARRIERS

EFFORTS TO CHANGE POLICIES MAY FAIL

As mentioned earlier, policy change may take a long time; unfortunately, sometimes efforts will fail. Last minute compromises, a change of administrators, unexpected events, newly elected officials, and changes in levels of support from key constituencies, can all result in a failure to make policy changes. Obviously, this can be frustrating and discouraging. Practitioners will need to be patient, maintain a long view, and keep up their efforts.

Many of the modern epidemics such as cancer and HIV/AIDS are manifested over years and decades. Perseverance is a necessity because most new initiatives are not adopted the first time they are considered. For example, when dealing with advocacy groups and elected officials, a longer-term communication strategy may be needed to infuse the process with new energy over months and even years.

STRUCTURAL AND ROLE CHANGES

Changes in the legislative arena (e.g., term limits) and other leadership changes (e.g., the rapid turnover of state health officers) may influence the timing and intensity of efforts to work with policy makers. Another challenge for administrators is the rapidly changing landscape in public health and in the delivery of health care. The growth of managed care and movements of many public health agencies away from direct service delivery have made the ability to anticipate and deal effectively with change even more crucial. Because of these ongoing changes, turnover of policy makers (especially administrators) is common; public health practitioners need to maintain their awareness of these changes in organizational structures, roles, and individuals.

ACTUAL OR PERCEIVED RESTRICTIONS ON LOBBYING

Related to the preceding discussion of organizational climate, practitioners may work in an environment in which there is institutional resistance to attempting to influence policies. For example, employees at mid- or lower levels of an organization such as a state pub-

TABLE 7.4 – SUGGESTIONS FOR COMPOSING A LETTER TO AN ELECTED OFFICIAL

Do not use a form letter
Cover only one topic or issue
State the purpose at the outset
When possible, provide cost impacts
Identify yourself and your organization
Enclose applicable editorials, data fact sheets, or position papers
Ask your policy maker for a response
If applicable, provide a courtesy copy to your organization
Thank your policymaker for his/her cooperation
When applicable, describe legislation by its bill number
Be polite/give reasons for support
Include recipient's name and address on both envelope and letter
Write legibly or type
Send a note of appreciation if and when the issue is supported

lic health department may have official or unofficial restrictions on policy or advocacy efforts related to their programmatic areas. Careful review of organizational or legal statutes is important, as the perception and reality of what constitutes lobbying is often at variance.

LACK OF LOCAL DATA

The presence of reliable data for small area analyses (e.g., a rural county or a legislative district) often does not exist, and this may lead to frustration among administrators and policy makers. Increasingly, public health agencies are aware of the need for more extensive and timely small area data.[25]

SUMMARY

Policy makers represent a critical communication audience for public health practitioners. This is because such persons make key decisions about laws, organizational practices, regulations, programs, and resources that can have substantial impact on the health of the public. Effective communication of public health data to key policy makers is a challenging task, and must be done in a manner that is clear, articulate, and inspiring using scientific information and data strategically.

As when communicating with other nonscientific audiences, practitioners must have a clear understanding of the purpose, audience, and message for the communication. Persuasion is usually the purpose behind communicating with policy makers. Policy makers are busy people who make many decisions, so preparation and a clear and well-articulated message are needed. Maintaining the focus of the message, getting quickly to the point, using numbers appropriately, avoiding jargon and clichés, being concise, being specific, and using real world examples are the best means of reaching both elected officials and administrators. When communicating with elected officials, other recommendations include understanding the legislative process, anticipating the arguments of the opposition, developing strong relations with elected officials, working with legislative staff members, and taking a long view towards policy change.

Success in effecting policy change is more likely to happen with multi-disciplinary approaches. Effectively conveying a body of public health information to an elected official may require teamwork from health communication specialists, managers, epidemiologists, and health educators. Networking among voluntary agencies, advocacy groups, and private agencies can provide an effective synergy. The ongoing revolution in information technology presents new opportunities for presenting public health information to policy makers. Practitioners must become proficient at understanding these new communication opportunities, but not lose sight of the ongoing importance of interpersonal interactions, such as face-to-face meetings and correspondence, when trying to communicate with these key individuals.

CHAPTER 7 ENDNOTES

1. Brownson RC, Newschaffer CJ, Ali-Aborghoui F. Policy research for disease prevention: challenges and practical recommendations. *Am J Public Health.* 1997;87:735-739.
2. Milio N. Priorities and strategies for promoting community-based prevention policies. *J Public Health Manage Pract.* 1998;4:14-28.
3. Schmid TL, Pratt M, Howze E. Policy as intervention: environmental and policy approaches to the prevention of cardiovascular disease. *Am J Public Health.* 1995;85:1207-11.
4. Goldman LK, Glantz SA. The passage and initial implementation of Oregon's Measure 44. *Tobacco*

Control. 1999;8:311-322.

5. Oregon Health Division. *Tobacco Prevention and Education Program Report 1999.* Portland, Oregon: Oregon Health Division, Department of Human Resources; 1999.

6. Brownson RC, Bal DG. The future of cancer control research and translation. *J Public Health Manag Pract.* 1996;2:56-64.

7. Shriver M, De Burger R, Brown C, Simpson HL, Meyerson B. Bridging the gap between science and practice: insight to researchers from practitioners. *Public Health Rep.* 1998;113(suppl. 1):189-193.

8. Institute of Medicine, *The Future of Public Health.* Washington, DC: National Academy Press; 1988.

9. Brownson RC, Simoes EJ. Measuring the impact of prevention research on public health practice. *Am J Prev Med.* 1999;16(3S):72-79.

10. Yankauer A. Science and social policy. *Am J Public Health.* 1984;74:1148-1149.

11. Wallack L, Dorfman L, Jernigan D, Themba M. *Media Advocacy and Public Health.* Newbury Park, CA: Sage; 1993.

12. Brownson RC. Epidemiology and health policy. In: Brownson RC, Petitti DB, eds. *Applied Epidemiology: Theory to Practice.* New York: Oxford University Press; 1998:349-387.

13. Sederburg WA. Perspectives of the legislator: allocating resources. *MMWR.* 1992;41(Suppl):37-48.

14. Scutchfield D, Keck W (eds). Principles of Public Health Practice. Albany, NY: Delmar Publishers; 1997.

15. Spasoff RA. *Epidemiologic Methods for Health Policy.* New York: Oxford University Press; 1999.

16. Sawicky M, ed. *The End of Welfare?: Consequences of Federal Devolution for the Nation (Economic Policy Institute Series).* Armonk, NY: ME Sharpe; 1999.

17. Tengs TO, Adama ME, Pliskin JS, Safran DG, Siegel JE, Weinstein MC, Graham JD. Five-hundred life-saving interventions and their cost-effectiveness. *Risk Analysis.* 1995;15:369-90.

18. Centers for Disease Control and Prevention. Consensus set of health status indicators for the general assessment of community health status—United States. *MMWR.* 1991;40:449-451.

19. Lengerich EJ, ed. *Indicators for Chronic Disease Surveillance: Consensus of CSTE, ASTCDPD, and CDC.* Atlanta, GA: Council of State and Territorial Epidemiologists; 1999.

20. Bier VM. On the state of the art: risk communication to decision-makers. *Reliability Engineering and System Safety* 2001;71:151-157.

21. Davis K. *Medicaid: The Health Care Safety Net for the Nation's Poor.* Testimony before the Committee on Finance, The United States Senate, Hearing on Welfare and Medicaid Reform, June 19, 1996. New York: The Commonwealth Fund.

22. Davis JR, Schwartz R, Wheeler F, Lancaster RB. Intervention methods for chronic disease control. In: Brownson RC, Remington PW, Davis JR, Eds. *Chronic Disease Epidemiology and Control.* 2nd ed. Washington, DC: American Public Health Association; 1998.

23. Liang AP, Renard PG, Robinson C, Richards TB. Survey of leadership skills needed for state and territorial heath officers, United States, 1988. *Public Health Rep.* 1993;108:116-120.

24. Boedigheimer SF, Gebbie KM. Currently employed public health administrators: Are they prepared? *J Public Health Manag Pract* 2001;7:30-36.

25. Figgs LW, Bloom Y, Dugbatey K, Stanwyck CA, Nelson DE, Brownson RC. Uses of behavioral risk factor surveillance system data, 1993-1997. *Am J Public Health.* 2000;90:774-776.

SUGGESTED READINGS AND RESOURCES

Brownson RC, Kreuter MW. Future trends affecting public health: challenges and opportunities. *J Public Health Manage Pract.* 1997;3:49-60.

Milio N. Priorities and strategies for promoting community-based prevention policies. *J Public Health Manage Pract.* 1998;4:14-28.

Sederburg WA. Perspectives of the legislator: allocating resources. *MMWR.* 1992:41(suppl):37-48.

Spasoff RA. *Epidemiologic Methods for Health Policy.* New York: Oxford University Press; 1999.

Stroup DF, Teutsch SM, eds. *Statistics in Public Health. Quantitative Approaches to Public Health Problems.* New York: Oxford University Press; 1998.

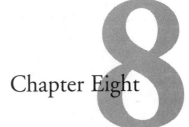

Chapter Eight

COMMUNICATING PUBLIC HEALTH INFORMATION TO PRIVATE AND VOLUNTARY HEALTH ORGANIZATIONS

Patrick Remington, MD, MPH
David Ahrens, MA

One goal of public health is to encourage organized community efforts by providing information on the health of the public and on effective policies and programs.[1] To achieve this goal, public agencies must work closely with voluntary, professional, or advocacy organizations in their communities.[2,3] The focus of this chapter is on how public health agencies can collaborate when information is communicated by public health agencies to private and voluntary health organizations in efforts to communicate public health information. Although written from the perspective of a public health agency, these strategies may be useful to any organization interested in improving the health of the public through coordinated community efforts.

BACKGROUND

Public health information is central to their mission, for many of these voluntary health organizations. For example, the American Cancer Society reports trends in cancer incidence and mortality in their "Cancer Facts and Figures" to emphasize the public health burden from cancer.[4] Similarly, a statewide AIDS coalition may report AIDS surveillance data to bring attention to the need for more prevention and intervention resources among high-risk populations.[5]

Public health professionals may achieve their communication objectives targeted to policy makers or the general public by working with private and voluntary organizations (Figure 8.1).[6] These organizations can influence the health of the public in several ways. First, they may lobby elected officials in support of health-promoting laws, programs, and public policies. In this regard, they perform a function that governmental public health agencies may not be able to perform. Second, they are able to enact private health policies within their own organizations that promote health; a managed care organization's decision to include smoking cessation as a standard benefit is an example of such a policy. Finally,

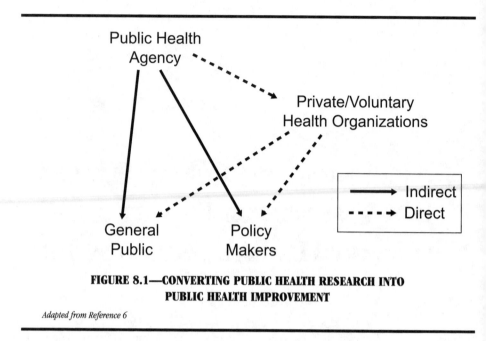

**FIGURE 8.1—CONVERTING PUBLIC HEALTH RESEARCH INTO
PUBLIC HEALTH IMPROVEMENT**

Adapted from Reference 6

these organizations often communicate directly with the public or through health care providers, either to provide information or to motivate health behaviors.

TYPES OF PRIVATE AND VOLUNTARY HEALTH ORGANIZATIONS

The words "public health" are often equated with activities performed by governmental public health agencies.[7] However, it is arguable that the programs and policies of private, non-governmental, and voluntary health agencies determine the health of the public as much (or more) than those of governmental public health departments. These organizations can be considered to fall into two broad categories: private health organizations or voluntary health organizations. Examples from each type of organization are included in Table 8.1. Note that some voluntary organizations concentrate more on advocacy while others have a greater focus on education and other services for their members.

PRIVATE HEALTH ORGANIZATIONS

Private health organizations include those organizations involved along the full spectrum of health care. These include employers who purchase health insurance, health insurance companies, managed care organizations, hospitals, and multi-specialty clinics. These organizations have taken an increasing interest in public health initiatives as they consider ways to improve the health of their members and patients and reduce excess health care costs. These initiatives may include everything from classes in weight loss and stress reduction to financial incentives to health care providers who provide high-quality, low-cost heath care. A second type of private organization involved in public health issues is a professional society or association. Examples include the American Medical Association and the affiliated county and state medical societies; nursing, pharmacy, or dental associations, or the American Public Health Association and its state affiliates. These organizations often develop and promote health policies on behalf of their members and actively engage in continuing professional education. In addition, they often lobby for public policies that support their organizational goals.

VOLUNTARY HEALTH ORGANIZATIONS

Voluntary health organizations have played a long-standing role in public health initiatives. Historically, voluntary health organizations such as the American Cancer Society, American Heart Association, or American Lung Association, had an educational focus and provided clinically relevant information on diseases to the public and health professionals alike. More recently, several voluntary health organizations have recognized the important role that public policies play in public health. With this increased awareness has come a shift from the traditional educational focus to a greater focus on engaging their members to advocate for certain public policies on health issues, and to lobby elected officials.

A volunteer board of directors often shapes the content of the educational and advocacy efforts. These boards are comprised of citizens with interest in the health issue, often as a result of either being affected by a health condition (e.g., cancer), or by having a family member with the disease.

RATIONALE FOR COMMUNICATING INFORMATION TO PRIVATE AND VOLUNTARY HEALTH ORGANIZATIONS

Why should a public health department collaborate with communicate health information to private and voluntary health organizations in health communication efforts? The transcript of a workshop given at Philip Morris' 1984 Corporate Affairs World Conference provides some important insights on working with third parties to achieve credibility, power, access, and leverage.[8] The speaker says that to be successful, Philip Morris had to be

---

TABLE 8.1—EXAMPLES OF PRIVATE AND VOLUNTARY HEALTH ORGANIZATIONS

Private Health Organizations
Professional organizations or societies (e.g., medical, nursing, pharmacy, public health, dental)
Health care providers
Health Maintenance Organizations (HMOs)
Health insurance companies

Voluntary Health Organizations
American Association of Retired Persons (AARP)
AIDS Action organizations
Alliance for Mentally Ill
American Cancer Society
American Heart Association
American Lung Association
Child Abuse Prevention
Farm Safety Organizations
March of Dimes
Multiple Sclerosis Society
Refugee service organizations
SIDS organizations
Tobacco-free organizations
United Cerebral Palsy

willing to ". . . put things together in fact to invent things that didn't exist before, coalitions, associations, institutes, seminars, meetings, all kinds of things like that. Example: the self-extinguishing cigarette. Who would normally be involved in the self-extinguishing cigarette on the other side of the fence? Probably the fire-fighting community. As you know, in the United States we have put a huge amount of time into helping all the organized groups of professional and volunteer fire fighters. They get such help from us that it is monumental. And then when we need them to stand up and say, (that it is) not cigarettes that cause fire in 99.9 percent of cases, we get their cooperation. But that is because we have cultivated them, helped them achieve some of their goals and we have seen that they are a potential enemy that has real credibility."[8]

Like Philip Morris, public health organizations can increase the likelihood of achieving their objectives by developing strategic community collaborations and partnerships. Public health agencies are often the source of "bad news" about health, including issues such as death, violence, sex, or drug use. Because of the controversial and often political nature of these issues, employees of public health agencies may find themselves constrained from presenting public health information in the most effective manner. Even in instances when a public health agency can directly communicate certain types of information, agency staff may recognize that there are other organizations better positioned to present the information to help achieve their overall communication objective.

INCREASED LEGITIMACY AND CREDIBILITY OF MESSAGES

While a public health agency may have substantial credibility in one sphere of activity such as disease prevention, it may not be as credible as a society of health professionals with a specific mission, such as the local chapter of the American Academy of Family Practitioners. The "specialization" of the organization generally implies a higher level of expertise and communications from these organizations and may receive greater recognition and prominence from the news media and public.

This perceived expertise may translate into a higher level of responsiveness among specific populations. For example, a news story featuring the state's pediatric medical society discussing the high incidence of lead poisoning may be more likely to win the attention of a legislator than a story originating within a public health agency. In addition to an organization's own members, professional health organizations have broad constituencies that add credence and legitimacy to their communications because of their history, expertise, or membership.

To better "drive home" the point of a specific report or study, a public health organization may seek an individual, such as a local professor or other expert, to present public health information. A similar role can be played by a leading volunteer or officer of a related organization (from a local hospital or health professional organization, for example), since these individuals are viewed as credible experts outside of the agency reporting the information.

MESSAGES ORIGINATING WITHIN ORGANIZATIONS RESONANT BETTER WITH MEMBERS

One of the features of private and voluntary health organizations is their specialization in areas such as lung disease, heart disease, kidney disease, cancer, or minority health issues. Members of these organizations contribute time and money out of a unique concern.

When leaders of such organizations speak, members usually listen. Also, private and voluntary health organizations often have employees who provide newsletters, bulletins, or electronic communications to their members, and are able to feature the story in a more detailed print-version for this highly interested group.

OPPORTUNITY TO INFLUENCE THE POLITICAL PROCESS

Public and private health organizations have vastly different relationships to the political and governmental decision-making process. Public health agencies are in the executive branch of government. As such, they have the advantage of a wide array of access to decision-makers within government, but they may be unable to communicate effectively certain types of essential information to the general public. For example, many public health agencies have historically been constrained from broadly publicizing morbidity and mortality related to use of tobacco or firearms because of the political power of tobacco and firearm interests in their jurisdictions.

Some public health agencies may also be substantially restrained or entirely barred from communicating with elected officials. In the past, this was limited to the state legislature, but the 1998 Federal Acquisition Streamlining Amendment (FASA) has limited state health officials from lobbying local elected officials. In many jurisdictions, public health agencies must filter their communications through a central authority at the highest level of a government agency, and employees may be constrained by a political agenda of the administration that oversees their activities.

Private and voluntary health organizations are often less encumbered in their communications within the political process, especially when they separate their educational and advocacy activities from their service function. Thus, many organizations can engage openly in direct lobbying for legislation, policies, and appropriations. Personnel within private health and voluntary health organizations often have strong relationships with specific legislators because of personal or professional ties; a legislator may work closely with the state affiliate of the "Alliance for the Mentally Ill" as a result of personal experience with a family member with mental illness. While few private and voluntary health organizations engage in direct electoral activity, those who do are often powerful at the state and local level. Common examples include state medical societies, private hospital corporations, and state hospital associations, as these groups often have well-financed political action committees and extensive networks of influential constituents spread throughout the state.

INFLUENCE ORGANIZATIONAL DEVELOPMENT

Information is an important "product" of private and voluntary health organizations. These organizations must engage in a range of reliable communication activities to educate and win support for their mission, but few organizations have the capacity to conduct such research. Public health agencies, through their programs and surveillance systems, are often the source of this information. Public health organizations can play an essential role in assisting local and state private health organizations to identify issues and develop communications that "connect" them to their membership and the public. Box 8.1 provides a specific example in one state.

BOX 8.1

The Wisconsin state medical society had identified tobacco use reduction as a major health priority and action item on its policy agenda. However, its attempts to involve members in its legislative activity on tobacco were limited because of a low level of interest within the organization on the issue. Seeing an opportunity to create an avenue for publication of research and to heighten the profile of tobacco-related issues among the membership of the medical society, a public health physician offered to solicit articles each year for an issue of their medical journal dedicated to tobacco. Over the next five years, numerous articles were published that highlighted the public health effects of tobacco as well as strategies for use reduction. Many positive effects can be attributed to the "annual tobacco edition." These included a significantly higher level of local tobacco control advocacy efforts by physicians (e.g., smoke-free public places), increased institutional involvement with other organizations involved in tobacco control legislative activities, and a higher level of perceived expertise in this area for its professional journal within the medical community and among the public. At the same time, the state medical society received substantial benefits for the annual issue. These tobacco-dedicated journal issues provided information to their members, particularly their younger members, on an issue of great concern to them. These journal issues also provided a positive connection between the medical society and the major public health concern of the public; each publication was accompanied by a series of press releases to increase press attention on tobacco issues and the work of the medical society.

PURPOSE, AUDIENCE, AND MESSAGE

Public health agencies often disseminate information "because it's there." These releases of data into a "policy vacuum" often receive scant attention from the news media, and rarely lead to positive action such as promoting a public health policy or changing behavior among the public. Granted, much of the communication of information from agencies to private or voluntary health organizations is in response to requests from these groups. To work proactively with these organizations, however, and to link information with action, a more planned and organized approach is needed.[9-11]

As described in chapter 2, practitioners need to define the purpose for communicating (why) and then identify a private or voluntary health organization (audience) that can assist them achieve their purpose. Is the primary purpose to inform or persuade, and is the information to be directed towards individuals or policy makers? More specifically, is the communication intended to increase public awareness about a certain health issue? Is it to change a specific behavior, such as reducing binge drinking or increasing the use of gun safety locks, or to promote passage of a certain policy, such as a mandatory seatbelt law or clean indoor air policy? The public health organization and the partnering private or voluntary health organization must together define the communication objective and the communication strategy.

The mission of these private and voluntary health organizations ranges from educating the public to grass roots policy advocacy. Messages that support the mission of an organization will be embraced by that organization. Virtually all major private and voluntary health organizations now have Internet Web sites that provide extensive information about their mission, operations, priorities, and personnel, and can be useful to public health professionals in identifying potential partners.

A simple and effective strategy for getting to know the mission and the staff of a voluntary health organization is to join it, as many voluntary health organizations are constantly looking for volunteers. Volunteers often begin working at the local level at city or county chapters. By working with the local staff and volunteers, practitioners can get to know the people, purpose, and culture of the organization. Most voluntary organizations have state level activities, such as planning committees or statewide public education efforts. Developing a close relationship with one or more key employees or volunteers in an organization will increase the likelihood of an effective partnership for communicating public health information.

The message—the specific information provided to private or voluntary health organizations—will vary widely and depend on the purpose for the communication, the organization, the topic, and the situation. Staff or members of voluntary or private health organizations may be highly trained, experienced health professionals or they may be people with limited expertise; nevertheless, it is essential that all parties agree on the central message and explicitly agree to adhere to it, especially if one party is asked to comment on the other's report.

SUGGESTED TYPES OF PUBLIC HEALTH DATA TO COMMUNICATE

Having public health data and other information that is pertinent to the mission of a private or voluntary health organization greatly increases the likelihood that the organization will communicate it widely. Although many types of health information can be communicated, the following categories are often of greatest interest to these organizations.

DISEASE BURDEN

Many voluntary health organizations have as their mission to reduce the burden from a particular disease; the American Cancer Society, American Diabetes Association, American Heart Association, or the March of Dimes are a few examples. Information from public health agencies that is likely to be most relevant to private health organizations are data that describe the public health burden from a relevant risk factor, condition, or disease.[12-19]

Public health burden can be measured in a variety of ways. These include (1) the number of deaths or years of productive life lost; (2) the use of health care services such as hospitalizations, emergency room visits, or ambulatory care visits and related costs; (3) the direct or indirect costs such as medical expenses, disability, or work days lost; (4) the number of people affected, prevalence rates, or incidence rates; or (5) the reduction in the quality of life.

Data on the burden of diseases and conditions is increasingly available electronically (see appendix 2 and 3). For example, mortality data since 1979 is available at no cost from CDC's Web site.[20] Similarly, many state health departments have put health data online for public use (appendix 3). Although relatively easy to access, practitioners in public health agencies can assist private or voluntary health organizations in the analysis and interpretation of such data.

TRENDS IN DISEASE OR RISK FACTORS

Private and voluntary health organizations and the public in general are interested in trends in diseases and health conditions. Increasing rates of disease or risk factors heighten public interest and often elicit a call for more prevention resources. Decreasing or unchanging rates may show the success of a public health campaign or help identify areas for continued emphasis.

The Healthy People Objectives, begun in 1990 and continued for 2000 and 2010, focused attention on the importance of setting objectives and carefully monitoring progress over time.[21] Many voluntary health organizations have adopted similar health outcome objectives. For example, the American Cancer Society set ambitious challenge goals for the American public for a 25% reduction in cancer incidence rates and a 50% reduction in cancer mortality rates by 2015.[22]

LOCAL RATES AND VARIATION

Just as "all politics is local," public health data is most useful at the local level. Recognizing the truth of this adage, private and voluntary health organizations regularly request health information at the county or community level. Local data make abstract problems more relevant to local decision-makers, and may help focus public attention on the issue at hand. For example, data on the increasing national incidence of breast cancer may receive some local attention and interest, but data showing higher than expected breast cancer incidence in a specific community engenders tremendous public attention and concern.[23]

If data are not available on the number of persons in the community with a certain condition, practitioners may be able to provide estimates using data from a referent population. For example, the prevalence of diabetes by age groups has been determined in national surveys. These age-specific rates may be applied to the population of a specific community to provide an estimate of the number of persons with diabetes.

Public health agencies at the state and national level, such as state health departments and the Centers for Disease Control and Prevention, may find that local public health agencies are better situated to communicate local public health data. For example, many state health departments have developed reports on the health of residents in specific areas in their states. These community health profiles are of great interest to private and voluntary health organizations at the state and local level and can be used to support community public health initiatives. Some states publish these profiles on their state health department Web pages and update them regularly. However, because of the nature of these detailed profiles, they tend to be ignored by the media and all but the most astute and engaged policy makers.

HEALTH DISPARITIES

Many private and voluntary health organizations conduct focused activities for special populations, such as the elderly, poor, minorities, or disabled. These organizations are often interested in data and other information that describe the health of their population of interest. Data that demonstrate disparities in health status, conditions, disease, or death rates may be especially valuable. Effective community intervention studies that affect relevant population groups are often also of great interest.

NEGOTIATING AN EXCHANGE

The collaboration of a public health agency with a private or voluntary health organization is more likely to succeed in achieving its objective and are more likely to help achieve the communication purpose and advance public health goals if there is a potential gain for both organizations. As described in chapter 2, the market concept of an "exchange" can be used to increase the effectiveness of health communications.[24] Just as the concept of exchange can be used to motivate individual behavior, an exchange can be negotiated to increase the chances of an effective health communication collaboration.

A private or voluntary health organization is often willing to assist a public health agency in achieving its goals if the organization's mission is to improve health. The communication objective will be more likely to be achieved if the public health information satisfies the needs and priorities of the private health organization. The organization's needs may include increasing public awareness of a health issue, providing useful information to members, raising money through contributions, increasing the stature of their organization in the community, using information to assist in grant writing, promoting a legislative issue, or increasing staff expertise.

Negotiating an exchange is usually straightforward when the private or voluntary health organization shares a mission closely aligned with the mission of the public health agency. Both agencies, for example, might have an objective to disseminate information widely to promote healthy behaviors (Box 8.2).

BOX 8.2

Tobacco is a leading cause of morbidity, mortality, and economic costs in a state. To document this burden, a state health department conducts a study to estimate the burden of tobacco in each county and in the state as a whole. The county data is especially helpful for local tobacco control efforts. To disseminate this information widely, the state health department provides the results directly to the state division of the American Cancer Society (ACS). In exchange, the ACS publishes a high quality report that includes the public health department's data on the burden of the tobacco. This report is widely distributed and the ACS logo is prominently displayed. Advocates throughout the state promoting the funding of aggressive tobacco prevention and control policies repeatedly use these local data from the ACS report over the next several years.

The mission of the American Diabetes Association is to prevent diabetes and diabetes-related complications through public awareness and research. Because they rely solely on contributions for their programs, they must have high visibility in the community. The state public health department has information about the burden of this disease in selected communities throughout the state (e.g., prevalence, hospitalizations, deaths, and estimated health care costs). The state chapter of the Diabetes Association is willing to produce a high quality publication, publicize the findings, and disseminate the information throughout the state, but the organization insists on having their logo prominently displayed on the cover of the document. The public health agency requests a one page acknowledgment in the front of the report citing the work of the agency staff members who collected and analyzed data used in the report.

Negotiating an explicit exchange improves collaboration and helps assure that each organization benefits and that information will be communicated more effectively and efficiently. A public health agency is more likely to achieve their goals if they are willing to share credit for the information with private or voluntary health organizations, leading to a "win-win" experience In practice, however, it is sometimes difficult for public health agencies to "give away" this information. Taking a backstage approach and letting others share the credit may be a two-edged sword, as it heightens the credibility and resources of the private health organization but provides the public health agency with little or no public recognition for its contribution. Over time, this lack of public visibility may leave the public health agency with little support from the public and policy makers.

CHALLENGES AND BARRIERS

Communicating public health information to private and voluntary health organizations

---

BOX 8.3

Infant mortality rates in a state have leveled off for the past several years. During a meeting of the statewide voluntary maternal and health coalition, one of the coalition members noticed that the infant mortality rate increased in the past year. He shares this with a health reporter at a major state newspaper, resulting in a front-page story proclaiming "infant mortality rates on the rise in state." This story leads to an active debate among policy makers; within a week a representative from an impoverished legislative district introduces a bill to increase funding for prenatal care programs for the poor. Meanwhile, epidemiologists at the public health agency conduct additional analyses and discover that the change in infant mortality was not statistically significant but simply reflected baseline variability around a level rate. In fact, more recently available (and unpublished) data demonstrate a continuing decline in the infant mortality rate.

---

can present difficulties, especially when the needs and interests of the public health agency conflict with those of the private or voluntary organization or when multiple organizations are involved.

CONFLICT OF INTEREST

The problem of a conflict of interest between a public health agency and a private or voluntary health organization can sometime occur; Box 8.3 provides an example.

This example presents a dilemma: should these data be used to promote a worthy program? Clearly the infant mortality rate did not increase but rather demonstrated random variability. A research scientist would say that this is a misuse and misinterpretation of the data. A community health advocate might justify the use of data, since it promoted a worthy and needed program. Some have suggested that there should be a distinct separation between science and policy.[25] In practice, public health practitioners must often bridge the gap between science and policy, but their credibility as an unbiased source of public health information will be compromised if they place advocacy ahead of science.[26,27]

MULTIPLE ORGANIZATIONS

Difficulty may arise when multiple private or voluntary health organizations share the concern about a specific topic and are interested in an agency's public health information. This issue arises often when communicating with the news media, as different organizations compete to get information first and create an "exclusive" story. There are a few diplomatic approaches for addressing the potential problem of private or voluntary organizations competing for information.

One way is to apportion the findings between the organizations so that each organization can issue its own report. Just as with the news media, questions will inevitably arise as to which organization gets the most "savory" data. Another approach is for the federal, state, or local public health agency to encourage collaboration between organizations. If the organizations have never worked together or jointly created a news release, this presents an important opportunity to build bridges. Never underestimate the importance or difficulty of negotiating these collaborations, however; issues such as whose logo is in the middle or the top of the page or who speaks first at the press conference can be very difficult to negotiate. If these strategies fail and the public health agency must choose to work with only one of the organizations, then the ability to communicate effectively, proximity and resonance to the larger audience, history of working with a public health organization, and other contributions are important considerations.

SUMMARY

Private and voluntary organizations are important audiences for public health information for the purpose of informing or persuading individuals and policy makers. Because governmental public health staff are often precluded from lobbying elected officials, sharing health information with private and voluntary agencies permit others to accomplish this goal. Efforts to communicate will be more effective if public health professionals decide on the purpose of the communication, understand the private or voluntary organization, and negotiate an equitable exchange for that information. Safeguards must be in place to assure that information is not misused and to avoid potential conflicts between public health agencies and private organizations.

The increasing recognition of the importance of health information has led to changes in some private and voluntary health organizations. Some organizations have hired epidemiologists to obtain, analyze, interpret, and disseminate public health data. Others have added additional organizational capacities that permit them to influence public policy directly, overcoming limitations on lobbying by not-for-profit organizations. Improving collaboration between public, private, and voluntary health agencies will improve the likelihood that public health communication goals are met.

CHAPTER 8 ENDNOTES

1. Institute of Medicine. *The Future of Public Health.* Washington DC: National Academy Press; 1988.
2. Nelson JC, Rashid H, Galvin VG, Essien JD, Levine LM. Public/private partners. Key factors in creating a strategic alliance for community health. *Am J Prev Med.* 1999; 16 (suppl 3):94-102.
3. Halverson PK, Miller CA, Kaluzny AD, Fried BJ, Schenck SE, Richards TB. Performing public health functions: the perceived contribution of public health and other community agencies. *J Health Hum Serv Adm.* 1996;18:288-303.
4. Wingo PA, Ries LA, Giovino GA, et al. Annual report to the nation on the status of cancer, 1973-1996, with a special section on lung cancer and tobacco smoking. *J Natl Cancer Inst.* 1999;91:675-90.
5. Hoxie NJ, Vergeront JM, Davis JP. AIDS and HIV in Wisconsin: projections for the decade. *Wis Med J.* 1990;89:261-6.
6. New York Academy of Medicine. *Medicine & Public Health: The Power of Collaboration.* New York, NY: Division of Public Health, New York Academy of Medicine; 1997.
7. Sommer A. W(h)ither public health. *Public Health Rep.* 1995;110:657-61.
8. Blake J, Dowling J, Florio D, et al. Workshop dealing with issues indirectly: constituencies [transcript]. September 13, 1984. Philip Morris document Web site (http://www.pmdocs.com/PDF/2025421934_2000.PDF). Date of access: June 6, 2002.
9. Remington PL, Goodman RA. Chronic disease surveillance. In: Brownson RC, Remington PL, Davis JR, eds. *Chronic Disease Epidemiology and Control.* 2nd Ed. Washington, DC: American Public Health Association;1998.
10. Remington PL. Communicating Epidemiologic Information. In: Brownson RC and Petitti DB, eds. *Applied Epidemiology.* New York: Oxford, 1998.
11. Goodman RA, Remington PL, Howard RJ. Communicating information for action. In: Teutsch SM, Churchill RE, eds. *The Principles and Practice of Public Health Surveillance.* New York: Oxford; 1994.
12. Remington P, Lantz P. Obesity in Wisconsin. *Wis Med J.* 1990;89:172,174,176.
13. Peterson DE, Akgulian NA, Remington PL. Alcohol-related disease impact in Wisconsin, 1988. *Wis Med J.* 1990;89:232-4,236.
14. Moss ME, Remington PL, Peterson DE. The costs of smoking in Wisconsin: a silent epidemic. *Wis Med J.* 1990;89:646,648,651.
15. Sleath B, Remington P. Increasing incidence of end stage renal disease in Wisconsin: 1982-1990. *Wis Med J.* 1992;91:303-4.
16. Remington PL, Stahlsmith L, Nashold R. Assessing the increase in firearm-related homicides in

Wisconsin, 1979-1993. *Wis Med J.* 1995;94:27-9.

17. Chudy NE, Remington PL, Blustein J. The costs of traumatic spinal cord and brain injuries in Wisconsin. *Wis Med J.* 1995;94:147-49.

18. Watson L, Yoast R, Wood S, Remington PL. The costs of cigarette smoking to Wisconsin's Medicaid program. *Wis Med J.* 1995;94:236-238.

19. Ford L, Remington PL. The burden of diabetes: the cost of diabetes hospitalizations in Wisconsin, 1994. *Wis Med J.* 1996;95:168-70.

20. Centers for Disease Control Web site. Available at: http://www.cdc.gov.

21. U.S. Dept of Health and Human Services. *Healthy People 2010.* Washington, DC: US Department of Health and Human Services; 2000.

22. Byers T, Mouchawar J, Marks J, et al. The American Cancer Society challenge goals. How far can cancer rates decline in the U.S. by the year 2015? *Cancer.* 1999;86:715-27.

23. Remington PL, Park S. Breast cancer incidence and mortality in Milwaukee's North Shore communities. *Wis Med J.* 1997;96:46-7.

24. Rothschild M. Carrots, sticks, and promises: a conceptual framework for the management of public health and social issue behaviors. *J Marketing.* 1999;63:24-37.

25. Rothman KJ, Poole C. Science and policy making. *Am J Public Health.* 1985;75:340-341.

26. Wallack L. Media advocacy: a strategy for empowering people and communities. *J Public Health Policy.* 1994;15:420-436.

27. Wallack L, Dorfman L. Media advocacy: a strategy for advancing policy and promoting health. *Health Edu Q.* 1996;23:293-317.

SUGGESTED READINGS AND RESOURCES

Goodman RA, Remington PL, Howard RJ. Communicating information for action with the public health system. In: Teutsch SM, Churchill RE, eds: *The Principles and Practice of Public Health Surveillance, 2nd ed.* New York: Oxford; 2000.

Remington PL. Communicating epidemiologic information. In: Brownson RC and Petitti DB, eds: *Applied Epidemiology.* New York: Oxford; 1998.

Remington PL, Goodman RA. Chronic disease surveillance. In: Brownson RC, Remington PL, Davis JR, eds: *Chronic Disease Epidemiology and Control.* 2nd ed. Washington, DC: American Public Health Association;1998.

Rothschild M. Carrots, sticks, and promises: a conceptual framework for the management of public health and social issue behaviors. *J Marketing.* 1999;63:24-37.

Wallack L, Dorfman L, Woodruff K. Communications and public health. In: Scutchfield FD, Keck W, eds. *Principles of Public Health Care Practice.* Clifton Park, NY: Delmar; 1996.

PART III:

MESSAGE DELIVERY

Chapter Nine

WRITTEN COMMUNICATION

Patrick L. Remington, MD, MPH
Lee Ann Riesenberg, RN, MS
Dianne L. Needham, MPA, PE
Paul Siegel, MD, MPH

Written communication is indispensable to the process of public health. Text in written form is the foundation for a wide array of communication options used in the public health domain. Writing enables the communicator to transmit information through time and across large distances without distortion. Because of writing's quasi-permanent nature, most people are motivated to confirm the accuracy of what they write to a greater degree than what they say.

BACKGROUND

The vast majority of public health communication tools originate in written form. Whether these tools manifest as electronic text, video and audio clips, or printed health education booklets, each demands sharp attention to the writing. Written communication performs a wide variety of functions, including informing audiences about health matters, persuading health policy makers, and telling the stories of science and medicine.

This chapter provides an overview of written materials commonly used in public health. Descriptions of, purposes for, and strategies on how to develop various written communication pieces for the general public and government legislators are presented. The intent and scope here is not to teach writing but to emphasize the importance of considering the details of writing.

TYPES OF WRITTEN MATERIALS USED IN PUBLIC HEALTH COMMUNICATION

Public health information can be written for nonscientific audiences in various formats, including technical, educational, and special reports (Table 9.1). Traditional public health information, such as vital statistics or disease surveillance, is often conveyed in technical reports that are rarely appropriate for nonscientific audiences.

TABLE 9.1—TYPES OF WRITTEN PUBLIC HEALTH COMMUNICATION PRODUCTS

Product	Primary Audience
Technical Reports and Publications	
Scientific publications (e.g., journal articles)	Public health professionals, Health
Annual reports	care providers
Surveillance reports	
Chart books or atlases	
Educational Reports	
Fact sheets	General public, News media,
Flyers/brochures/pamphlets	Health care providers, Voluntary
Tailored print communication	health organizations, Private
Question and Answer (Q&A) sheets	health organizations
Frequently Asked questions (FAQs)	
Posters	
Press releases	
Special Reports	
Plans	Policy makers
Proposals	
Policy assessments	
Legislation-related materials	

By contrast, educational and special reports focus more on specific types of information, and aim at communicating information for a specific purpose. Descriptions of the characteristics and contents of these reports follow.

TECHNICAL REPORTS AND PUBLICATIONS

The bulk of technical reports—such as scientific publications, annual reports, surveillance reports, chart books, and atlases—are primarily written for public health professionals or health care providers. Specific examples include journal articles; routine reports on cancer registries, infectious diseases, or managed care organization performance (e.g. Health Plan Employer Data and Information Set [HEDIS]); and other reports such as Health United States 2000, Healthy People 2010, Consensus Development Statements, and Surgeon General Reports.

These technical reports represent official opinions and recommendations, rigorously standardized and researched. They are usually read in a targeted manner—rather than cover-to-cover—by readers who may scan a selected section or two seeking an informed and authoritative answer to a specific question for use in making a personal or policy decision. Such documents are sources for the development of other, more concise written materials.

Public health information is sometimes presented in scientific publications, such as state medical society or applied public health journals. These reports follow the specific guidelines of the journal, and are often reviewed by editorial staff and peer reviewers.

Clearly written executive summaries or abstracts are especially important if information is to be reviewed and understood by policy makers. Summaries need to be carefully crafted to highlight the key points and recommended action steps. However, as noted in the next section, technical reports are not well-suited for communicating targeted messages to the general public or policy makers.

EDUCATIONAL REPORTS

Public health practitioners have historically created materials written to educate or inform the general public or policy makers. Primarily designed for individual health promotion efforts, the general public is nearly always the main audience. Examples of educational reports include fact sheets, flyers, brochures, pamphlets, tailored print communication, question and answer sheets (Q & A), frequently asked questions (FAQs), posters, and press releases. The Wisconsin Department of Health and Family Services Diabetes Control Program, for example, has developed a number of written materials. These include *Essential Diabetes Mellitus Care Guidelines, Diabetes Facts for Wisconsin, Year 2000 Wisconsin Public Health Agenda: Diabetes-Related Goals, Partners in Diabetes Prevention,* county maps showing the burden of diabetes in Wisconsin, and a diabetes resources guide.[1]

Fact sheets, flyers, brochures, and pamphlets usually contain a small amount of background information, the main message, and a readily accessible resource for obtaining further information.[2] Brochures, pamphlets, and press releases in contrast to the shorter-format items (fact sheets, flyers, Q & A sheets, and FAQs), are usually folded, using a four- or six-panel design format to display key points with bullets, bolded text, or larger font sizes. Readability and interest are improved by the creative use of white space and graphics (e.g., clip art, photographs, or color).

Tailored print communication refers to materials intended to reach a specific targeted audience. Messages are based on the unique characteristics of that audience, are related to the desired outcome, and are derived from an individual assessment.[3] Tailored print communication takes into account the attitudes, perceptions, and behaviors of the specific individuals.[4] Examples of tailored print messages may include stressing the financial benefits of quitting smoking or addressing perceived barriers to mammography.[3] Tailored messages are usually developed through computer-generated algorithms, and are increasingly delivered via electronic communication (chapter 12).[3,5] There is some evidence that tailored print messages are more effective than generic print materials for health education and behavior change.[3,4,6,7]

Press releases are one- or two-page written documents that target the print, broadcast, and online news media. They are written to relay newly released information, such as a health statistics report or scientific study; key points are highlighted and a comment or two from relevant officials may be included. Media relations professionals routinely create press releases. Working with news media representatives is discussed further in chapter 6.

SPECIAL REPORTS

Special reports are commonly written for a specific audience or purpose, and many are designed for advocacy; by their very nature, advocacy materials are written in a proactive voice. Policy makers may occasionally request that public health agencies develop such documents to plead, argue, or provide active support in favor of a cause, idea, or policy. Examples may include needs assessments, policy assessments, strategic plans, action plans, position papers (commonly referred to as white papers), program funding proposals, as well as "action sheets" that emphasize recommended policy actions or a need for program resources.

A policy assessment provides a scientifically justified basis for a position or evaluates the pros and cons of several positions in question. Policy assessments are, in effect, scientific papers with appropriately referenced citations and appendices and a short executive summary. In contrast to a policy assessment, Position papers, on the other hand, attempt to explain the need and rationale for a particular policy and are generally only a few pages in length. In contrast to a policy assessment, a position paper is usually targeted to a nonscientific audience, and may include numeric analogies or statements such as "the tobacco industry recruited 'a classroom a day' of school children to replace smokers lost to death or quitting in a given state." Public health program proposals provide a formal description of how a potential program would be conducted and its attendant costs.

Finally, there are several types of written materials designed specifically for elected officials: these include legislative testimony, proposed legislation, and implementation language. Written materials for legislators are covered in chapter 7; creating proposed legislation and implementation language is rarely done by public health practitioners and is beyond the scope of this book.

PURPOSE, AUDIENCE, AND MESSAGE

Understanding the purpose, audience, and message are crucial to developing appropriate and effective written materials. Determining the essential 'why and who' for the written communication product are often overlooked first steps. Information is regularly released without considering whether the goal is to inform or persuade an audience; for example, a report describing the burden of diabetes in a community is meant primarily to educate, while a newspaper opinion-editorial (more commonly called op-ed) or letter-to-the editor intends to persuade readers. Sometimes a written piece has a dual role—a state report on cancer may both educate the general public and persuade policy makers to increase funding for cancer control activities. As with other types of communication, written materials may be developed reactively or proactively, depending on the situation and audience.

After determining the purpose and audience, the communication message must be developed. Depending on the issue and circumstances, this may consist of simply providing written data to raise awareness or it may require a persuasive letter to an elected official recommending policy changes. Accurate assessment of an intended audience's level of knowledge is at the core of message development. Public health professionals who develop communication messages often forget that their main audience may not have the appropriate level of knowledge and understanding of the issue(s). As a result, practitioners should be aware of the scientific literacy level of their intended audience and carefully and simply explain the scientific terms and concepts.

Written materials should be pre-tested, whenever feasible, before they are widely distributed. Pre-testing the accuracy of the scientific content should be done with other public health experts, and with members of the intended audience for general comprehension and format appeal. This is especially true when developing written materials intended for use by the general public, as such materials are commonly written at reading levels that are too high.[8] (Writing for low literacy audiences is discussed later in this chapter.)

GENERAL RECOMMENDATIONS FOR WRITTEN COMMUNICATION

Although many forms of written communication exist, certain principles are applicable to public health communication. These include brevity and highlighting key points, leveraging material for different audiences, and effectively organizing information. A discussion of each of these general considerations follows.

BE BRIEF AND HIGHLIGHT KEY POINTS

With the large amount of information available in multiple formats, there is a tremendous need for brevity in communication products. The corporate world has long acknowledged the need for brief, to-the-point communications; in fact many companies adhere to a one-page maximum length for internal communication tools.

As shorter written communication products are preferred and expected, practitioners must learn to write to the point. This means applying a good writing style such as using active verbs, introducing the important message and recommended actions quickly, and highlighting key message facts. Techniques for highlighting text include use of lists, bullets, bolded texts, and larger font sizes.

LEVERAGE INFORMATION FROM LENGTHY REPORTS OR RESEARCH STUDIES

Information from longer reports or scientific studies may be translated or "leveraged" into shorter written products tailored to specific nonscientific audiences. This is most evident in the use of press releases; a number of scientific journals routinely provide releases to reach both scientific and nonscientific audiences.

Practitioners in both government and non-government positions often readily adapt information from longer reports and scientific studies into educational reports such as fact sheets, brochures, pamphlets, and newsletters. Sometimes information from longer reports can also be adapted for advocacy reports such as position papers or funding proposals.

Official government reports are routinely screened at higher organizational levels, enabling government agency staff members to adapt the material into new formats to reach specific audiences. People in non-governmental positions can also readily adapt government reports, as such reports are not subject to copyright restrictions.

For research studies, a three-tiered leveraging approach works well, with one report written for the broad scientific audience (e.g., scientific journal article); a two- to four-page report or newsletter geared toward public health practitioners or health care providers; and a one-page fact sheet or pamphlet for the general public.

Using templates designed for specific audiences can standardize leveraged reports. A state health report, for example, could contain information about childhood immunization that is appropriate for all counties within that state. Another approach is to use a template that could be developed for a series of reports for each county, targeting local public health practitioners; each report would include similar text but would use county-specific data.

ORGANIZE THE INFORMATION

Written material must be well organized to be effective. Information, whether for technical, educational, or special reports, needs to be arranged in a logical sequence familiar to the intended audience.

Written material may be organized into one of five major formats for presentation to nonscientific audiences. The selected format depends on the purpose, audience, and details of the communication situation.

Chronological order, such as summarizing past events or requesting future actions to occur within a certain time order

Order of importance, such as describing items or details from most-to-least important

Cause and effect, which is a variation of chronological order but emphasizes the cause followed by the effect(s)

General to specific, which starts with a general information summary or request, followed by specific details relevant to the summary or the request

Pros and cons, used to present information by covering both sides of an issue

SPECIFIC RECOMMENDATIONS FOR WRITTEN COMMUNICATION

Creating high quality written materials for public health communication that are brief and tailored to specific audiences is difficult. The following content and style recommendations (Table 9.2) can assist practitioners in their writing efforts.[9]

CONTENT RECOMMENDATIONS

When writing for nonscientific audiences it is essential to communicate a few main points. This means minimizing text to suit the short amount of time audiences will devote to reading the information. The main points should also be repeated in the introduction, body, and conclusion of the communication product.

TABLE 9.2 - SPECIFIC RECOMMENDATIONS FOR IMPROVING WRITTEN COMMUNICATION

Content
- Include no more than three or four main points
- Repeat main points
- Develop an interesting point of entry
- Provide examples and use analogies
- Explain complex terms and relationships
- Minimize use of numbers
- Acknowledge health misconceptions and opposition arguments
- Use culturally appropriate language
- Assess literacy levels
- Consider tailoring the message to match audience needs

Style
- Use "Plain English" and avoid jargon
- Use active voice (verbs)
- Use appropriate tone
- Keep sentences and paragraphs short
- Consider adding graphics
- Use attractive layout and design

Adapted from Reference 9

Since many readers skim written text, the introductory section must grab their attention. Headlines, subheadings, short quotations, graphics, and sidebars are all important points of entry for attracting the readers' initial attention (Box 9.1).[10] The first few sentences are also critical; human-interest stories, anecdotes, or quotations can help to attract readers and create interest.[11]

Analogies and examples help convey and maintain reader interest, particularly for the general public, news media, or elected officials. Analogies can help readers understand complex public health topics by linking complicated subjects to something they are already familiar with. Describing the size of a heart in congestive failure as "big as a grapefruit" compared to a normal heart that is the 'size of your fist' can help most audiences better understand certain health facts.

Use of simple words is preferred in written communication, but sometimes more complex terms are required. If this is the case, then new terminology must be introduced slowly and be thoroughly explained, for example, 'mainstream smoke is the smoke drawn through the mouthpiece at the end of the cigarette.'[12] Similarly, complex relationships need to be introduced and presented in as simple terms as possible, often one step at a time.

Use of data should be kept to a minimum. One or two meaningful numbers are likely to be much more effective than a series of statistics. Communication goals can address pre-

---

BOX 9.1

Human profiles and science sidebars were used extensively in a comprehensive diabetes research plan that was prepared for and presented to Congress. This sidebar illustrates how such text creates greater reader appeal in an essentially technical document.

Pam Fernandes
"My first ride on the tandem came about when I worked in community relations at the Massachusetts Association for the Blind. A fellow phoned in wanting to volunteer to take a blind person out on his tandem bike. The call was connected to me simply because I worked out in the gym. I'm blind and people thought I might know where to refer him. When I suggested various programs, he said he'd already been in contact with them but that they weren't doing anything currently, and he wanted to ride now. I told him I'd be glad to oblige. We got together, did a 20-mile ride and I loved it.

I'm going into my seventh season of tandem bicycle racing. In my very first race I came in last but I have progressed. Since then I've won four national championships and two international medals. One of the international medals is the Bronze from the 1996 Paralympic Games in Atlanta and the other is the Silver from the 1994 World Championships for Disabled Cyclists in Belgium...

There are a lot of reasons why I race. For me, it has turned into a platform to demonstrate ability and teach other people through my example. When I'm tandem cycling the true disability is not my blindness; the true disability is the diabetes. If you are blind, once you get used to it, all you have to do is get a tandem bike and find partners who ride. This isn't easy but it's "doable" and consistent—you can ride with the same guy every Wednesday on the same bike. With diabetes, every day is a new day. Too many different things can affect your blood sugar that are difficult to balance and that make it really tough...

The best part of having diabetes is being forced to understand nutrition and how our bodies utilize energy. I have a disease where I have to pay attention to those things so I'm a much healthier person. The worst part about diabetes is losing people to it—unnecessarily in some cases—and experiencing the complications of the disease."

Adapted from reference 10

existing misconceptions or opposition arguments. One way to deal with misconceptions or opposition arguments is to state them clearly, acknowledge how and why they may seem to make sense, describe the flaws, and provide a better explanation.[13]

Finally, use culturally appropriate language if materials are intended for minority populations.[14] Text should be directed to the most specific group(s), whenever possible: Mexican-Americans as opposed to Hispanics, for instance. When preparing such materials, advice from leaders of the appropriate group(s) or organization(s) can be invaluable.[14] If materials are to be translated into another language, the translator must have experience with the intended group, and back-translation (translating text in the new language back to English) should be used to identify errors.[14] Pre-testing translated communication material with the intended audience is an essential step in such efforts.

STYLE RECOMMENDATIONS

Use "plain English" and avoid jargon when communicating with nonscientific audiences. The Plain Language Action Network[15] has established three principles to follow in developing user-friendly government documents:

Use reader-oriented writing—write for the customers, not for other government employees

Use natural expression—as much as possible, write as one speaks, and write with commonly-used words in the way they are naturally used

Make the document visually appealing—present the text in a way that highlights the main points

Substitute simple, short words for multisyllable words, such as "poor" not "substandard," "clotting" or "thickening" not "coagulation." Table 9.3 provides examples of converting technical or complex health terms into language better understood by nonscientists. At times using a technical word is necessary either because there is no other term or because readers will need to learn it for future reference in the written product. When this occurs, a definition or description of the technical term is required at first use.

The active voice, or use of active verbs, greatly improves readability.[16] For example, the passive voice in the phrase "A decision was made to. . . " should be changed to "Officials at the X County Health Department decided to. . . ." The passive voice can usually be converted to the active voice by asking the question, "Who did what?" In some situations using the passive voice is appropriate; for example, "James Watson was awarded the Nobel Prize for discovering the molecular structure of DNA."

Sentences and paragraphs should be kept as short as possible, especially when communicating with the general public. Many writers have a tendency to create lengthy sentences that are difficult to decipher. When explaining complex ideas, using several short and uncomplicated sentences can help overcome the problem of long sentences. Paragraphs should be kept short (e.g., limit each paragraph to five sentences) and address one main topic to attract and keep readers' interest.

Whenever possible, consider adding graphics to written materials. Photographs, diagrams, clip art, and simple charts can enhance text messages, improve comprehension and retention, and prevent reader fatigue.

TABLE 9.3—EXAMPLES OF TRANSLATING COMMON PUBLIC HEALTH TERMS TO SIMPLER LANGUAGE

Public Health Term	Simple Language
Acute	Lasting a short time
Advocacy	Help
Alternative	Different
Angina pectoris	Chest pain
Atrophy	Decreasing size, wasting away, shrinking
Cardiac	Heart
Cerebrovascular accident	Stroke
Conjecture	Guess
Correctional facility	Jail
Deficit	Loss, shortage
Demonstrate	Show
Determine	Find, find out, figure out
Enhances	Increases
End-point	Result
Etiology	Cause
Facilitate	Ease, help
Interface	Talk, discuss
Gastrointestinal	Stomach, food track
Health care facility	Clinic or doctor's office
Idiopathic	Unknown cause
Impact	Effect
Initiative	Effort
Lipid	Fat
Occupational	Work-related, job-related
Occlude	Close off
Optimum	Best
Physician	Doctor
Postpartum	After childbirth
Pulmonary	Lungs
Recommendation	What we suggest, what you should do
Subsequent	Next, after, later
Surveillance	Observation, monitoring, watching
Thrombus	Blood clot
Uterus	Womb
Utilize	Use
Vascular	Blood vessels
Vertigo	Dizziness

WRITING FOR LOW LITERACY AUDIENCES

Literacy is an important determinant when preparing written materials for the general public.[8] Based on findings from a 1992 national survey, 47% of the adult population have marginal reading skills, and fully 21% of all adults read at or below a fifth grade level.[17] Projected nationally, more than 90 million individuals have limited ability to read, comprehend, or act on what they read. This makes highly readable materials essential for reaching general public audiences.

Readability refers to the ease with which the text can be understood, and is usually referred to in terms of the equivalent school-grade level. There are at least 40 systems designed to estimate readability of materials.[18] In general, readability levels are calculated based on the length of words (syllables) and the number of sentences in the text. The systems most commonly used are the Flesch, Fog, Fry, and SMOG indexes.[19] Table 9.4 details two examples of written materials from a health care setting that were revised to lower reading levels.[8] Despite the dramatic reduction in reading grade level, the materials are not simplistic. Shortening sentences, adding graphics, and highlighting important items is especially important for low literacy audiences to read and retain the information.

Readability indexes do have their drawbacks. There is variability and lack of comparability for readability systems,[19-22] and reading comprehension is often two to three years below reading levels based on these indexes.[19] One study found that the average patient reading level is almost five years lower than the last grade of school completed.[23] Special care should also be exercised when making use of the readability indices that are available through commercially packaged word processing software.[8]

Table 9.5 lists the factors that can improve readability for low literacy audiences:[8] related words or phrases need to be grouped together and presented in a logical sequence; short bulleted lists and boxes containing key points are often helpful for grouping and sequencing; short and familiar words, and short sentences, are essential. As described in the previous section, using the active voice improves writing, and personal pronouns (e.g., we or you) help engage the reader.

Vivid nouns, verbs, and phrases should be used. Concrete examples (rather than abstract principles) with specific recommendations about actions to take greatly increase writing clarity and effectiveness. Finally, the tone of writing is also important. An instructional or invitational tone, such as, "we need to work together to . . ." or "here's how you can help . . .", can draw the reader in.[8] Pre-testing materials with members of the intended audience can help identify major problems and ways to improve the final product.

SUMMARY

The overarching goal when communicating public health information in writing is to say what needs to be said in the fewest words possible. Writing a lengthy technical report with information for health professionals may be easier, but it will be less effective than developing educational or advocacy materials to persuade policy makers or the general public to behave a certain way.

Technical, educational, and special reports are the primary forms of written communication products in public health, and each category typically targets one or more nonscientific audience. Knowing the purpose, audience, message, and preferred communication channel for the intended audience will enhance the quality of written materials. These

TABLE 9.4—EXAMPLES OF REVISED TEXT FOR LOW LITERACY AUDIENCES

Example 1: Poison Ivy

Original Text: 9th Grade Reading Level

Poison ivy, poison oak, and poison sumac plants can cause a severe skin reaction when their leaves come in contact with human skin. The result of the contact with one of these plants is a red, bumpy skin rash, usually on areas of the body where the skin is thinnest, like the arms, shins, and face. There may be swelling near the rash, which usually progresses to itchy blisters that ooze, harden and then crack. What determines how soon a person reacts after exposure is how sensitive he or she is to the plant and the number of previous times the person has been exposed to it.

Most cases of poison ivy, oak, or sumac can be cared for at home and do not require a trip to a doctor. However, a small percentage of people are highly allergic. If you break out in a rash within 4 hours of exposure and your eyes swell shut and blisters form, seek medical attention immediately.

Revised Text: 4th Grade Reading Level

(Photograph or Diagram of Poison Oak, Poison Ivy, and Poison Sumac)

When your skin touches one of these leaves, your skin may react. What happens to your skin:
- red, bumpy skin rash
- swelling near the rash
- rash may be itchy and ooze
- usually occurs on arms, legs, and face
- as the rash heals, it may harden and crack

Some people are very allergic to these plants, while others are not allergic to them. Two things contribute to the severity of your skin reaction. People with sensitive skin may develop more of, or a worse rash. Also, if you have had a rash from one of these plants in the past, your skin may react more severely. Most of the time you can take care of your rash at home. However, if the rash is severe, you should see a doctor.

Reasons to see a doctor immediately:
- If you develop a rash or blisters very soon after you touch the plant
- If your eyes swell shut

Example 2: Prenatal Care

Original Text: 12th grade level

It makes good sense that premature births and newborn illnesses decrease with early pregnancy care. The doctor is actively involved in testing the pregnant woman for pregnancy-induced diabetes and a host of other problems that would not be detected by the patient alone. We know that these problems cause premature births and illnesses in newborns. It certainly makes sense that early detection and treatment of these problems by the doctor results in healthier babies.

Revised Text: 8th grade level

If you are pregnant or think you may be pregnant, call for an appointment right away. Getting care early in your pregnancy will help you have a healthy pregnancy and a healthy baby. Your Primary Care Physician (or an OB-GYN doctor you choose from our network) will give you a complete checkup. He or she will also give you certain tests to make sure everything is going well. If there are any problems, it's good to find them early. That way, you have the best chance for a healthy baby.

Revised Text: 4th grade level

If you are pregnant or think you might be, go to the doctor as soon as you can. If you start your care early, things will go better for you and your baby. Your own doctor or a childbirth doctor from our list will give you a first exam. Tests each month or so will let you know if all is going well.

If there is a problem, you will know right away. Then we can do what is needed. Early care is the best way to have a healthy child. Your baby counts on you.

Source Reference 8.

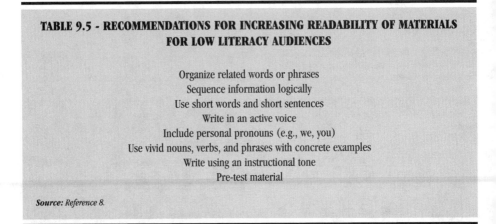

TABLE 9.5 - RECOMMENDATIONS FOR INCREASING READABILITY OF MATERIALS FOR LOW LITERACY AUDIENCES

Organize related words or phrases
Sequence information logically
Use short words and short sentences
Write in an active voice
Include personal pronouns (e.g., we, you)
Use vivid nouns, verbs, and phrases with concrete examples
Write using an instructional tone
Pre-test material

Source: Reference 8.

materials should be brief, well-organized, and highlight the key points of more lengthy technical reports or scientific studies.

The content and style of each communication piece should be tailored to the specific audience with, consideration given to the group's educational, socioeconomic, and cultural background. Writing for low-literacy audiences, which includes a large portion of the general population, can be especially challenging. Readability indexes, use of short words and sentences, writing in an active voice, and using personal pronouns and descriptive words are all keys to successful writing for such audiences. Throughout the process of preparing written materials, practitioners should pre-test messages with members of the intended audience.

Writing will continue to play a critical role in the ability to articulate public health information. As people are inundated with information in their daily lives, traditional written materials may be left behind unread. Practitioners must pay careful attention to producing written products that grab and hold readers' attention, are easy-to-read, and provide essential information quickly.

CHAPTER 9 ENDNOTES

1. Wisconsin Department of Health and Family Services Diabetes Control Program Publications. Available at: http://www.dhfs.state.wi.us/health. Date of access: March 14, 2002.
2. United States Department of Health and Human Services Press Releases. Available at: http://www.hhs.gov/news/press/2002.html. Date of access: July 7, 2002.
3. Kreuter MW, Strecher VJ, Glassman B. One size does not fit all: the case for tailored print materials. *Ann Behav Med.* 1999;21:276-283.
4. Rimer BK, Glassman B. Is there a use for tailored print communications in cancer risk communication? *JNCI Monograph.* 1999;25:140-148.
5. Kreuter MW, Farrrell D, Olevitch L, Brennan L. *Tailoring Health Messages: Customizing Communication Using Computer Technology.* Mahway, NJ: Erlbaum; 1999.
6. Skinner CS, Campbell MK, Rimer BK, Curry S, Prochaska JO. How effective is tailored print communication? *Ann Behav Med.* 1999;21:290-298.
7. Revere D, Dunbar PJ: Review of computer-generated outpatient health behavior interventions: clinical encounters "in absentia". *J Am Med Inform Assoc.* 2001;8:62-79.
8. Root, J., Stableford S. *Write It Easy-to-Read: A Guide to Creating Plain English Materials.* Biddleford,

ME: Maine AHEC Literacy Center; 1997.

9. Gastel, B. *Presenting Science to the Public*. Philadelphia, PA: ISI Press; 1983.

10. Needham D. Personal profile of Pam Fernandes. In: *Conquering Diabetes: A Strategic Plan for the 21st Century*. Washington, DC: Congressionally-Established Diabetes Research Working Group, 1999, pages 36-37.

11. Gastel, B. *Health Writer's Handbook*. Ames, IA: Iowa State University Press, 1998.

12. United States Department of Health and Human Services, Substance Abuse and Mental Health Services Administration. *Reducing Tobacco Use Among Youth: Community-Based Approaches*. DHHS Publication No. (SMA) 97-3146l; 1997.

13. Rowan, K.E. Strategies for explaining complex science news. *Journalism Educator*. 1990; 45:25-31.

14. Centers for Disease Control and Prevention. *Scientific and Technical Information Simply Put: Tips for Creating Easy-to-Read Print Materials Your Audience Will Want to Read and Use*. 2nd ed. Atlanta, GA: Centers for Disease Control and Prevention, Office of Communication; 1999.

15. Plain Language Action Network Web site: http://www.plainlanguage.gov. Date of access: July 7, 2002

16. Strunk, W., White, E.B. *The Elements of Style*. 4th ed. Boston: Allyn & Bacon; 2000. New York, NY: Macmillan, 1979

17. Kirsh IS, Jungeblut A, Jenkins L, Kolstad A. *Adult Literacy in America: A First Look at the Results of the National Adult Literacy Survey*. Washington, DC: U.S. Department of Education; 1993.

18. Davis, T.C., Crouch, M.A., Wills, G., Miller, S., Abdehou, D.M. The gap between patient reading comprehension and the readability of patient education materials. *J Fam Pract*. 1990; 31:533-538.

19. Bauman, A. The comprehensibility of asthma education materials. *Patient Education and Counseling*. 1997; 32:S51-S59.

20. Pichert J.W., Elam P. Readability formulas may mislead you. *Patient Educ Counseling*. 1985;7:181-191.

21. Meade C.D., Smith C.F. Readability formulas: Cautions and criteria. *Patient Education and Counseling*. 1991;17:153-158.

22. Klingbell, C., Speece, M.W., Schubiner, H. Readability of pediatric patient education materials: current perspectives on an old problem. *Clin Pediatr*. 1995; 34:96-102.

23. Jackson, R.H., Davis, T.C., Bairnsfather, L.E., George R.B., Crouch M.A., Gault H. Patient reading ability: an overlooked problem in health care. *Southern Med J*. 1991; 84:1172-1175.

SUGGESTED READING AND RESOURCES

Ad Hoc Committee on Health Literacy. Health literacy report of the Council of Scientific Affairs. *JAMA*. 1999; 281(6):552-557.

Berger AA. *Improving Writing Skills: Memos, Letters, Reports, and Proposals*. Newbury Park, CA: Sage; 1993.

Centers for Disease Control and Prevention. *Scientific and Technical Information Simply Put: Tips for Creating Easy-to-Read Print Materials Your Audience Will Want to Read and Use*. 2nd ed. Atlanta, GA: Centers for Disease Control and Prevention, Office of Communication; 1999.

Churchill E. *MOD:COMM—A Communications Module*. Atlanta, GA: United States Public Health Service, Centers for Disease Control and Prevention; 1994.

Doak, C.C., Doak, L.G., & Root, J.H. *Teaching Patients with Low Literacy Skills*. 2nd ed. Philadelphia, PA: J.B. Lippinicoatt, Williams & Wilkins Company; 1996.

Gastel B. *Health Writer's Handbook*. Ames, IA: Iowa State University Press; 1998.

Root J, Stableford S. *Write It Easy-to-Read: A Guide to Creating Plain English Materials*. Biddleford, ME: Maine AHEC Literacy Center; 1997.

Maggio R. *The Dictionary of Bias-free Usage: A Guide to Nondiscriminatory Language.* Phoenix, AZ: Oryx Press; 1991.

Maggio R. *Talking About People: A Guide to Fair and Accurate Language.* Phoenix, AZ: Oryx Press; 1997.

Schwager E. *Medical English Usage and Abusage.* Phoenix, AZ: Oryx Press; 1991.

Strunk W, White EB. *The Elements of Style*, 4th ed. Boston: Allyn & Bacon; 2000. New York, NY: Macmillan, 1979.

Chapter Ten

ORAL PRESENTATIONS

J. Gregory Payne, PhD

O ral communication has always been the primary form of human communication. Despite the development of new technologies such as the Internet, oral communication remains a primary means for communicating public health messages, and having effective oral presentation skills is a common job requirement in public health. Giving formal oral presentations, or public speaking, often generates much anxiety for speakers, however, oral communication skills can be learned by public health practitioners. The purpose of this chapter is to provide an overview of the principles of oral presentations and practical advice on developing and improving speaking skills for public health practice.

BACKGROUND

Oral communication is the oldest form of human communication, and is based on the premise that a person's attitudes, beliefs, and values are capable of change. Prior to the invention of the written word about 6,000 years ago, oral communication was the primary means of human communication for health and other matters.[1] This is not surprising, given the large part of the human brain dedicated to speech and hearing and the strong preference for humans to interact with each other through oral means.[2] Oral communication remains an essential skill for most practitioners, and both health care providers and patients consider such skills as essential for furthering understanding on health issues.[3]

Most oral communication activities are interpersonal (or dyadic), that is, they involve one-on-one information exchanges[4,5] such as in-person meetings, telephone calls, or distance-based visual technology. A second common form of oral communication is small-group communication, which is characterized by various leadership and participant roles.[6] The third type of oral communication is public communication, which is the focus of this chapter. Public communication consists of formal speaking (giving a speech) to audiences that can range from a single policy maker, to a national or international audience watching or listening on television, radio, or the Internet. The term "oral presentation" as used in this chapter refers to such formal speaking occasions.

Whatever the setting, the major aim of any oral presentation was first described by Aristotle and remains unchanged today: to give a speech that is direct, relevant, and personal to the intended audience.[7] What constitutes an effective oral presentation is often assumed to be based on the innate ability of the speaker, but in reality, the principles and practices of effective oral presentations are well-known and can be used to advance public health goals.

CHARACTERISTICS OF ORAL PRESENTATIONS

There are seven primary characteristics that underlie public speaking: purpose, audience, source (speaker), message, language and delivery, visual aids, and feedback.

PURPOSE

The first step for public health practitioners is to decide on the purpose (why) of the communication (chapter 2). Is the primary goal to provide information or to persuade individuals or policy makers to make certain decisions or take action? Is the presentation to be reactive or proactive? Because public health practitioners are often considered experts, the purpose of reactive oral presentations is usually to inform audiences; by contrast, the purpose of proactive oral presentations is generally persuasive: to encourage a change in individual behavior or beliefs or to encourage a change in a policy or for resource allocation, for example (Box 10.1). Oral presentations are commonly used for two other purposes: to inspire or to entertain audiences.[7,8] Such communications are much less commonly used by practitioners in work-related settings and are not covered in this chapter.

Persuasive communication is more difficult than informational communication. A persuasive oral presentation requires that the audience: (1) be informed about the issue; (2) trust the speaker; (3) be receptive to the information; (4) be open to a change in beliefs or action; and (5) have the capability or power to make a change.

BOX 10.1

The director of a health care purchasing cooperative in Madison, Wisconsin was interested in developing a community health improvement initiative. He brought together health care professionals from the local health plans and hospitals, business executives, public health professionals, citizens, and policy makers and formed a "Quality Forum." This group decided to focus their activities on addressing one or two health issues rather than diluting their efforts too broadly. To help decide on the key health issues to consider, they invited a public health practitioner from the state health department to address their group.

The practitioner gave a short oral presentation to the group. In the presentation, he opened with a discussion of the leading causes of death in the state. He discussed national estimates of the leading preventable causes of death,[9] then based on his own analyses, he presented the leading preventable causes of death in Wisconsin and provided reprints of a recent article on this topic.[10] As a result of the presentation, the Quality Forum decided to focus on tobacco use as a priority health issue. Over the next several years, the Forum implemented a collaborative project with the major health plans that attempted to increase the assessment of tobacco use among physicians. The group also developed a guide for businesses that described effective strategies and community resources for smoking cessation.

AUDIENCE

For an oral presentation, the specific audience is usually a group of people assembled in a specified place to receive a message from a predetermined speaker. As with all other forms of communication, understanding the audience's background, interests, and expectations (audience analysis or pre-speech evaluation) is essential.

Clearly, the purpose and message are integrally related to the specific audience, and practitioners need to learn as much as possible about their audiences and the context in advance to construct and deliver a speech effectively. Knowing the background of the event and the expectations of those sponsoring the presentation is essential, as each audience and speaking situation is unique.[5,7]

Audience analysis begins with the expected size of the audience, as well as demographic and other general characteristics (age, sex, education level, nationality, race/ethnicity, occupation, place of residence, geographic area, religion, political affiliation). Preparation, message development, language and delivery, audiovisuals, and audience interaction are likely to be quite different when presenting to one policy maker compared to presenting to several hundred people in a large conference room. Similarly, presentations to teenagers usually differ from those given to the elderly.

Audience analysis also consists of ascertaining if the audience has pre-existing knowledge, beliefs, and attitudes about the topic and if they have certain expectations about the speaker and the message. If an audience is well-versed about a specific health issue, then lengthy background descriptions and definitions are likely to be counterproductive. Understanding pre-existing beliefs and attitudes will help speakers determine if the audience will be hostile, neutral, or friendly. Closely related to audience characteristics is knowing where the speaker will appear on the agenda. Is this the only speech? Will other speakers precede or follow the presentation? If so, what is the expected purpose and focus of their remarks?

Finally, speakers need to remember that their presentations may reach unintended audiences. Given the advances in technology, messages delivered to a particular audience may also be broadcast by television, videotape, video-conferencing, or the Internet to other unintended ("invisible") audiences. Such media offer unparalleled access, but can have ramifications on a speaker's credibility if these audiences are not carefully considered when preparing and delivering remarks.

SOURCE (SPEAKER)

The source, or the speaker, refers to the role of image or ethos on oral communication. What is ethos? According to Golden, it is a qualitative assessment by the audience of the speaker's: (1) character or trustworthiness; (2) knowledge and expertise; (3) use of good will; and (4) charisma.[7,11] Ralph Waldo Emerson summed it up best: "What you are speaks so loudly, I can't hear what you say".[12] It has long been recognized that a speaker's ethos is the single most important factor in persuasive oral communication and has an enormous effect on the response by audiences to his or her message.[5,11,13] This is not surprising, given that in most oral presentations the speaker is directly visible, the presentation is live, and there is the opportunity for direct visual and audio interaction between the presenter and the audience.

The first component of ethos consists of character, or perceived trustworthiness, of the presenter. Listeners measure or respond to what is perceived to be a speaker's intent, as well as his or her overall reliability and sincerity. Public health practitioners are usually perceived to have high levels of trustworthiness because of their job titles and educational background, which can be enhanced or negated by past performance in a particular role. It is important to be honest when making oral presentations because if credibility is lost or damaged, it can be difficult or impossible to regain. Also, when a gap exists between what speakers say versus what they do, speakers lose much of their persuasive force. For instance, a morbidly obese individual is likely to be perceived by most audiences as a poor spokesperson for discussing the benefits of nutrition and physical activity.

The second ethos factor is expertise. The perceived expertise of a speaker has been found to increase audience interest and knowledge gained from oral communication.[5] For practitioners, perceived expertise is associated with their employer, job title, position within an organization, educational degrees, experience, or workplace success. As with character, public health practitioners are usually perceived by audiences to be experts.

The third characteristic of ethos is the degree of identification and good will between the speaker and audience. A speaker should try to identify with the audience by demonstrating that he or she understands something about their interests, needs, or concerns. This may be considered as courtship: an effective speaker needs to woo an audience.[11] Initial attempts to identify with an audience should occur in the opening or introduction of a speech. Too often public health practitioners (and scientists in general) ignore the need to identify with audiences at the very beginning of the speech by using even the simplest of techniques such as commenting on the weather, a major sports activity, a current news item, or another shared commonality discovered during audience analysis. Failing to identify with the audience, or worse, being too forceful, sarcastic, negative, or uncompromising can cause unnecessary ill will that can interfere with the receipt of the message.

The fourth characteristic of ethos is charisma. Charisma may be the result of a speaker's abilities, image, style, or life experience. A charismatic speaker may be one who has had a powerful personal health experience or problem and has overcome the problem or used it as a motivating force for action (such as a parent who has lost a child to a drunk driver). Charisma assumes two distinct forms: the audience bestows god-like qualities upon the speaker that elevate him or her to a higher level (very unusual in public health), or the audience is positively swayed and strongly identifies with the speaker because of his or her rhetorical power.[14,15]

Ethos is a key, but often neglected, element in oral communication. Because most public health practitioners are perceived by audiences to be trustworthy and have expertise, improvements in oral presentations are most likely to occur by developing or improving good will and charisma. This can be done through the effective use of vivid examples that are highly salient to the audience, as well as through rhetorical expertise gained through numerous public speaking situations.

MESSAGE

After understanding the purpose and audience, the next step is message development. What is the main message that the communicator wants the audience to remember? A message should be characterized by strong arguments and compelling appeals, but it should also prevent the audience from "jumping to conclusions." It must be based on valid premises, generalizations with supporting data or examples, reliable and unbiased testimony, and a conclusion with an appropriate rationale and frame of reference. If a message is properly developed and emphasized it tends to make audiences content-centered, rather than person-centered—ideas take precedence over images. Well-presented messages can help bring people together, generate knowledge and understanding, solidify or modify existing values, and result in the audience taking specific actions.

The message is composed of three parts: opening, body, and closing.[8] The opening should begin with a simple greeting ("good morning" or "good afternoon" are usually sufficient) followed by something that will get the audience's attention. This can be done by posing rhetorical questions, quoting well-known persons, making provocative statements, telling a short story, or using a visual or audio aid. The opening also should include a brief preview of what the presentation will cover.

The body is where the key points are presented. In general, presenters should remember the Rule of Three Major Points for oral communication: (1) Preview the three major points; (2) Describe and substantiate the three major points; and (3) Summarize the three major points.

The closing should briefly review the salient points from the body of the message, embrace the commonality of the speaker and the audience, and charge the audience to take the next step(s) needed for success.[8] Finally, speakers should finish with a pause and say "thank you" to signal to the audience the presentation is over. Table 10.1 is an example of an outline of the message for an oral presentation on mammography.

TABLE 10.1—EXAMPLE OF AN OUTLINE FOR A PERSUASIVE SPEECH

Purpose	To persuade an audience that primarily consists of women who are aged 50 years or older of the importance of early and frequent screening for breast cancer
Introduction	• Open with a greeting that refers to the occasion and the group. • Introduce topic using a (rhetorical) question: "How many of you here today are over 50?" (Indicate that they don't have to hold up their hands—as a humorous way —to keep their true age a secret to colleagues.) "How many of you have had a breast cancer screening exam in the past year?" • State that "Today I am here to talk to you about the importance to you and your family and loved ones of an annual mammogram to screen for breast cancer." • Preview the points to be covered: (1) who is at risk; (2) what steps should be taken; and (3) the time to act is now—for both you and your family.
Body	• Begin with an attention-getting step: "Breast cancer is every woman's problem.It has happened to Betty Ford, Linda McCartney, and Olivia Newton-John, as well as to your friends and neighbors. It can be deadly, but it also can be cured if caught early." • Outline the steps involved in getting a mammogram. Explain the procedure and the time involved. Include visual aids to help describe the success of mammography for early breast cancer detection. • Challenge each member to schedule an exam, both for their own peace of mind and for that of their families. Evoke the emotional theme of responsibility to oneself, to family and friends; emphasize the importance of taking a proactive rather than a reactive approach to discovering this disease.
Conclusion	• End the speech by highlighting the responsibility of each person to either schedule a test or to remind their wives and female friends to have such a preventive procedure. Highlight the example of a positive role model (the specific example depends on the audience analysis) such as a prominent national or local celebrity. • State that "This is the best gift you could give to those you love and who love you." • Close with a reference to the group or occasion, then thank the audience for the opportunity to speak.

For persuasive speeches, the speaker should stress shared values, beliefs, and experiences in the introductory remarks to help develop trust. The types of evidence offered in support of controversial points must be carefully considered. Nevertheless, evidence by itself does not achieve persuasion—it is only part of a dynamic relationship that can enhance a speaker's credibility and increase his or her ability to change the minds and the behaviors of audience members. Effective persuasive speakers explicitly state their desired outcome in the message, rather than making suggestions or providing hints.

An additional requirement for persuasive messages is that they that arouse and sustain audience interest, either through emotional or logical appeals, examples or illustrations. For example, after stating a principle, theory, or method, the speaker may introduce personal and relevant examples (incidents, stories [anecdotes], or descriptions) that will illustrate key points. This can usually be done by presenting new information; countering commonly held beliefs; displaying photographs; through conflict/humor; or discussion of compelling scientific or historical facts. If personal examples or short narratives are used, they must be meaningful to the audience.

Public health data in oral presentations should be clear and impressive, and emphasize or clarify key points. If overused, they tend to overwhelm the major points and can confuse audiences, especially persons with low numeracy. To be most effective, data should be presented visually, when possible, using bar charts, maps, pie charts, or line graphs (chapter 11). Strong numeric analogies are especially useful in oral presentations (chapter 3), as they can help anchor one or two key points in the minds of audiences.[16]

Humor can be an effective tool if it is relevant to the message, but speakers must have a very good understanding of their audience and what the audience will consider to be funny. What is humorous to one audience can be offensive to another and practitioners should be cautious, as many speakers have suffered irreparable damage to their credibility by a spontaneous attempt at humor that backfired.

Finally, consider the impact of non-verbal messages. For example, to downplay the danger of a water supply erroneously reported to have been contaminated, a meeting with families at or near their homes would carry great persuasive influence and support the statement that there is no danger to residents.

Message development often poses a challenge for public health practitioners. Messages need to be relevant to nonscientific audiences, and they need to be translated into words that are easy for these audiences to understand. Practitioners commonly fail to gain and sustain the audience's attention through the use of stories, photographs, quotes, compelling facts, or personal examples, resulting in relatively bland or colorless messages. Although such additional material involves more preparation time, it is often the difference between an average and an excellent presentation.

LANGUAGE AND DELIVERY

Language and delivery are the next feature of oral communication, and along with audiovisual aids, constitute the message production and delivery step for an oral presentation.

Language There are several criteria to improve language clarity, style, and vividness in oral communication (Table 10.2).[17,18] Clarity is the first consideration. Language should conform to national usage standards, as not doing so will likely adversely affect a speaker's ethos. Recognize that words are symbols and that meanings may differ. Depending upon

TABLE 10.2—LANGUAGE RECOMMENDATIONS FOR ORAL PRESENTATIONS

Conform to current national usage standards
Be aware of multiple meanings, context, and symbolism
Use conversational words and phrases
Use concrete rather than abstract or general words
Avoid jargon and technical terms
Use links and transitions
Avoid emotional distortions, superlatives, and exaggerations
Use similes and metaphors to improve vividness

the audience and the context (demographics and history), the perceived meaning of words to the audience may be quite different compared to their meaning to the speaker. Use words and phrases that are primarily oral in nature, that is, simple nouns and verbs commonly used in ordinary conversations. This makes presentations seem more informal, spontaneous, direct, and personal. Whenever possible, use concrete rather than overly general or abstract words. The overuse of jargon or highly technical language should be avoided,[19] and speakers should use appropriate verbiage for connecting links and transitions between different parts of the speech.

Language style is important in creating the proper atmosphere of the communication. Language filled with emotional distortions, superlatives, and exaggerations (idiot, fabulous, exciting, for example) is rarely appropriate, as terms with strong negative or positive connotations or excessive "zeal" can alienate and polarize audiences. The guiding principle is that the language be suitable for the speaker, the subject, and the occasion, with the goal to adopt a proper attitude that does not offend or create division.

Language vividness consists of using words to paint pictures in the minds of the audience, and it helps create presence and improve communion with the audience. This can be done by using figures of speech, similes, and metaphors. One example of this frequently used in anti-smoking campaigns is the contrast between the glamour once associated with smoking in advertisements and the horror of a model that contracted laryngeal cancer later in life and lost the ability to speak. Likewise, describing an ulcer as "like an open sore in the stomach" can help communicate the reason for pain to a non-medical audience.

Delivery A speaker's delivery plays a vital role in enabling audiences to receive and respond to the message, and consists of both verbal and non-verbal aspects (Table 10.3). Several factors are involved in creating an effective vocal pattern. A speaker's pitch (melody) helps to generate interest in a topic; the optimum pitch should be pleasing to the audience and the level should be varied–a monotone must be avoided as it makes audiences drowsy. Pronunciation refers to stress and accent on words or syllables, while articulation is concerned with syllable formation. The goal of good pronunciation and articulation is simply that the words be understood by the audience.

The rate, or timing of a speech, is also important. As a rule, most presenters need to concentrate on speaking slowly (anxiety usually makes people talk faster) and deliver the speech at a rate of no more than 120-140 words per minute. The use of filler sounds and words such as "er," "uh," "you know," "ok" (excessive vocalization) need to be avoided as they are distracting and reduce a speaker's credibility. Projection (force) refers to the voice loudness or intensity level; in many situations, a public address system is needed to ensure that

---

TABLE 10.3—DELIVERY RECOMMENDATIONS FOR ORAL PRESENTATIONS

Verbal Considerations
  Vary voice pitch or melody (avoid speaking in a monotone)
  Pronounce and articulate words and syllables
  Speak slowly
  Avoid filler sounds and words ("er," "uh," "you know," "ok")
  Project voice
  Use pauses or changes in voice level to stress key points

Nonverbal Considerations
  Wear conservative clothing and avoid adornments
  Look at the audience
  Interact with visual aids
  Avoid clutching or leaning on the podium
  Use gestures and movements appropriately
  Avoid distracting mannerisms (e.g., drinking water, hands in pockets, twirling a pen)

---

speakers are heard. Again, high anxiety levels often reduce vocal force; as a result, most speakers must focus on speaking louder (projecting their voices). Pauses or changes in voice projection (raising or lowering voice loudness) at the beginning, during, or at the end of a speech can be effective ways to stress key points; however, if they are used too frequently or at inappropriate times, they can become diversions or impediments.

Because of the in-person interaction between a speaker and the audience, the 6 major non-verbal aspects of oral communication are critical, yet often unrecognized, components of message delivery. The identification sought by the speaker with his or her audience is enhanced with the proper dress and appearance. A speaker's clothing should generally mirror that of the audience; distinctive clothing or adornments that garner attention (bright colors, extravagant patterns, hats, necklaces, pendants, campaign buttons, dangling earrings) should be avoided as they detract from the message. For most communication situations with nonscientific audiences, practitioners should plan to dress conservatively. For men, this means dress slacks, long sleeve shirt, a tie, and sometimes a sports coat; for women this means a dress or a blouse and skirt. Advanced research about the audience will help ensure proper dress, but when in doubt, it is best to dress more formally.

Eye contact helps improve the interactive nature of the communication and increases the perceived trustworthiness of the speaker. Presenters should look directly at the eyes of a listener and talk to those eyes, rather than rapidly scanning the audience. If visual aids are used, speakers need to routinely refer to key points on slides or overheads (through the use of a pointer). If the speaker is behind a podium, he or she should not clutch or lean on it; generally, speakers should keep their hands at their sides while speaking.

Hand or arm gestures, if used to emphasize key points and are not overdone, add life to a presentation. With wireless microphones now widely available, it is acceptable for speakers to occasionally move away from the podium. Mannerisms and activities such as placing hands in pockets, drinking from a glass, or fiddling with pens should be avoided as they are distracting.

VISUAL AIDS

Visual aids used with oral presentations include overheads, slides, computer graphics, videotape, and direct access to Internet Web sites. Using visual aids is strongly recommended for most speaking situations to nonscientists, as they can enhance delivery, are expected by most audiences, and improve audience retention of information.[20-22] To be effective, visual aids must provide essential additional information, support the message, and be interesting to the audience. A thorough discussion of visual communication is included in chapter 11. Audio-only aids such as music and audiotapes are much less commonly used for oral presentations in public health and are not covered in this chapter.

Table 10.4 lists the key elements for creating and using visuals. The physical layout and available equipment will determine whether visuals can be used. The room must have proper acoustics, sight lines (to avoid obstructed views), lighting, electrical outlets, and projecting equipment. To maintain clarity, each slide should have a single focus, and generally no more than one slide per minute should be used to prevent overuse and avoid overshadowing of the speaker's verbal message.

To improve readability, text should be minimized (<40 words per slide) by using short phrases, bulleted lists, and "white space."[23] To ensure maximum readability, font sizes need to be large (at least 24 point), and color combinations should have high contrast. Audiences usually have difficulty maintaining interest with text-only presentations, so practitioners should consider adding graphics, pictures, graphs, cartoons, etc. (chapter 11).

In addition to interacting with their slides, speakers should explain or describe the information on each slide. Visual overkill, that is, using too many slides or fancy software features, should be avoided as it creates unnecessary distractions and may reduce speaker credibility. Finally, back-up materials such as written notes or overheads should always be available, as visual projecting equipment often works improperly or fails. Even if a speaker brings his or her own equipment, he or she should be surprised and relieved if it actually operates as expected.

FEEDBACK

Feedback from the audience is the final feature of an oral presentation. Feedback is the audience's method of informing the speaker how the message is being interpreted or appreciated and constitutes the evaluation of the communication (chapter 2). Feedback for oral presentations is primarily non-verbal; eye contact (or lack of), arched eyebrows, folded arms, smiling, nodding of the head, spontaneous laughter, yawning, restlessness, talking,

---

TABLE 10.4—USE OF VISUAL AIDS FOR ORAL PRESENTATIONS

Consider physical layout and equipment
Include a single focus per slide
Use no more than 1 slide per minute
Minimize text on slides by using short phrases, bulleted lists, and open space
Minimize use of numbers
Use high contrast colors
Explain information on each slide
Avoid visual overkill
Prepare back-up materials

reading, or walking out of the room will communicate to the speaker the success or failure of the presentation.

Once the presentation is underway, the communicator must be constantly aware of audience feedback and make rapid adjustments to the message or delivery of the message, especially if the feedback is negative. Sometimes negative feedback is the result of external circumstances such as faulty audiovisual equipment, which should be corrected if possible. However, if negative feedback is the result of some other aspect of the delivery or the message itself, presenters must be prepared to adjust accordingly, such as shifting delivery methods, modifying messages, or changing or modifying the structure of arguments or evidence.

ADDITIONAL RECOMMENDATIONS FOR IMPROVING ORAL PRESENTATIONS

REHEARSE

Speaker preparation is directly related to effectiveness, and even the most renowned communicators rehearse their presentations. By rehearsing, speakers become intimately familiar with the message, timing, and audio-visual aids, and they can evaluate the overall presentation effectiveness. Familiarity and experience gained by rehearsing reduces speaker anxiety and makes the delivery more natural.

Rehearsal sessions should simulate the actual situation; if possible, rehearsals should occur in the planned location of the actual presentation (or a similar environment) and include audio and visual aids. Depending upon the speaker's experience and the importance of the presentation, videotaping, audiotaping, or rehearsing in front of a mirror can be helpful. Trial presentations should be done for colleagues or friends when possible. Such informal formative evaluation provides invaluable feedback to the speaker in helping to improve the message, language, delivery, and use of visual aids. In addition to rehearsing the presentation, speakers should anticipate and prepare answers to potentially difficult questions (discussed later in the chapter).

SPEAK EXTEMPORANEOUSLY

To insure a conversational and more natural delivery, presenters should speak extemporaneously, that is, use only an outline or notes. Reading presentations to audiences is strongly discouraged, as the sentence structure and vocabulary used in writing differs markedly from those used in conversation. Presenters who read speeches tend to speak in a monotone, have poor eye contact with the audience, and do a poor job assessing audience feedback. Presenters also should not memorize their material as again, this leads to a monotone delivery and poor ability to assess audience feedback.

EXAMINE THE SPEAKING ENVIRONMENT AND COMMUNICATION AIDS IN ADVANCE

It is common for the speaking environment to have some unexpected problems such as obstructed seating, poor lighting, and inoperable or absent equipment (microphones, pointers, visual projecting devices). Presenters should arrive at least 30 minutes early to allow ample time to examine the environment, test the equipment, and make adjustments prior to the arrival of the audience. If PowerPoint or 35-millimeter slides are used, they should viewed on the screen in advance to ensure that they are loaded properly.

PROVIDE WRITTEN HANDOUTS

Unless the audience is large, providing written handouts as adjuncts to oral presentations is recommended. They can be used to stress key points and to improve audience recall after the presentation has ended. With the advent of presentation software packages such as PowerPoint, creating written handouts is now easy to do. Generally, handouts should be passed out near the end or after a presentation; if disseminated earlier, they can rob the speaker of the attention of the audience.

STAY WITHIN THE TIME ALLOTTED

It is imperative that speakers present their material within the time that they have been allotted. Audiences almost always know how much time a given speaker has, and expect him or her to cover their material during this time period. Often the public health practitioner giving a presentation is one of several speakers, so common courtesy dictates staying within the time confines to be fair to others. To ignore time constraints can negatively affect the audience's evaluation of a speaker's ethos, not to mention upsetting fellow speakers. Sometimes the time allotted a presentation is reduced because of unanticipated events (equipment failure, fire alarm, a prior speaker or session taking more time than expected). When this occurs, speakers need to be adaptable to such situations and make adjustments to shorten, yet still cover, the key points of their presentations

RESPOND TO QUESTIONS

In many situations a speaker will be asked questions, and the following suggestions can improve question-and-answer dialogues with the audience (Table 10.5). Generally, issues raised by audience questions simply require further clarification; however, if the presentation covers challenging or controversial issues, speakers should anticipate difficult questions and be prepared with responses. Because most questions are spontaneous, audience members should be encouraged to ask them either during or immediately after the presentation. Repeating questions for the entire audience is strongly recommended: this ensures that the entire audience hears them, provides the speaker with a chance to restate questions and clarify any misunderstandings, and allows the speaker some time to develop answers.

Presenters should not refuse to answer a question. If there is a difference of opinion with a member of the audience, speakers should acknowledge it and move on. If a speaker does not know the answer, he/she can refer the question to a more knowledgeable person or

---

TABLE 10.5—RESPONDING TO QUESTIONS

Anticipate and prepare responses for potentially difficult questions
Allow questions either during or immediately after the presentation
Repeat questions
Do not refuse to answer
Take time to understand the question and develop a response
Be open and honest and do not project a defensive attitude
Maintain good eye contact with the questioner
Provide short, direct answers
Follow up if a response is deferred

defer a response and get back in touch with a questioner later. Presenters should carefully listen to questions and take the time to formulate an answer: pausing before answering is acceptable. Being open and honest in responding to questions is essential, and presenters should avoid a defensive attitude. If the presenter made a mistake that is pointed out by an audience member, he or she should admit it.

Good eye contact should be maintained with the questioner throughout the stating of the question and the response—it may help to consider the question and answer session as a one-on-one conversation occurring in a hallway or office. Responses to questions should be short and direct, as long-winded answers often fail to directly answer the question and can reduce the opportunity to entertain other questions. If the audience is the news media, presenters should strive to respond in quotable phrases or sound bites. Finally, as both a common courtesy and to maintain credibility, presenters must follow-up as soon as possible with audience members if they promise to provide answers or additional materials at a later time.

CHALLENGES AND BARRIERS

FAILING TO TAILOR PRESENTATIONS TO EACH AUDIENCE AND SITUATION

The biggest challenge faced by all speakers is tailoring presentations to the specific needs of each audience and situation. To reach audiences, practitioners should imagine themselves in their audience's shoes. To develop empathy with their audience, the speaker should translate messages to a personal level that identifies with the values of the audience, but tailoring goes far beyond audience analysis and message development. In each situation, practitioners must consider other aspects such as language, delivery, timing, visuals, and audience feedback.

For example, if a practitioner is making an oral presentation to a community group concerned about a chemical spill, he or she should acknowledge the audience's fear and anger before discussing statistics about risk. When presenting to an administrator or elected official, practitioners must recognize that such audiences generally concentrate on resource issues or political ramifications. Because of literacy or numeracy problems, presenting tables or mathematical models is likely to be ineffective with general public audiences.

PRESENTING TOO MUCH INFORMATION

A common mistake made by public health practitioners (and others) is to present too much information. Audiences cannot retain large amounts of information that is presented orally. Most oral presentations tend to be short (<20 minutes) and the best that most practitioners can do is to highlight a few main points in their message. The goal of a speech is not to provide the audience with all of the knowledge on a given topic; instead, it is to stimulate audience interest, understanding, or action.

MAINTAINING AUDIENCE INTEREST

With few exceptions, most public health practitioners are not natural entertainers, especially persons in more quantitative fields such as epidemiology or statistics. However, adding some vitality to presentations is essential to establish and maintain nonscientific audiences' interest. This is especially true for longer oral presentations. The use of relevant real world examples, humor, short stories, rhetorical questions, quotations, cartoons, videotapes, audiotapes, and photographs will improve the likelihood that audiences will attend to the message.

ADJUSTING WHEN PRESENTATIONS OCCUR AT INOPPORTUNE TIMES

Inevitably, there will be times when a practitioner must present at inopportune times. These include presenting just before a meal, late in the afternoon or evening, or after the audience has heard from a series of speakers. Inopportune times also occur when there is a concurrent event impacting the audience's attention (such as poor weather, fire alarm, political crisis, athletic event). In such situations, speakers need to adapt by preparing a short presentation that highlights their key points as quickly as possible. Humor may be useful in such situations.

SUMMARY

The major aim of any formal oral presentation is to give a speech that is direct, relevant, and personal to intended audiences. The 7 primary characteristics of oral communication for public speaking are purpose, audience, source (speaker), message, language and delivery, visual aids, and feedback. The purpose is the reason for the presentation, that is, deciding if the goal is to inform or persuade specific audiences. Persuasion is a common purpose for oral communication in public health. Audience analysis is closely related to the purpose and involves understanding the expected size of the audience; demographic characteristics; pre-existing knowledge, beliefs, and attitudes; and audience expectations for the speaker.

Trustworthiness, expertise, good will, and charisma are the four characteristics of the source (speaker), and are critical, but often overlooked, determinants of a presentation. The message contains the essential information the speaker wants the audience to remember, and consists of the introduction, body, and conclusion. As a rule, the message should contain no more than 3 main points. Language and delivery are the actual words and style of the presentation, and represent the how and where of oral communication. Visual aids are important adjuncts to presentations and are recommended in most situations. Feedback is the ongoing nonverbal and verbal clues provided by the audience to the speaker and the speaker to the audience during a presentation, and must be recognized and adapted to accordingly by both parties.

There are additional considerations for enhancing oral presentations. These include rehearsing, speaking extemporaneously, examining the speaking environment and communication aids in advance, providing written handouts, staying within the time allotted, and responding to questions. Failing to tailor presentations to each audience and situation, presenting too much information, maintaining audience interest, and making adjustments when presentations occur at inopportune times are common challenges.

Despite major advances in communication technology, the age-old art of public speaking, and the skills necessary to do so, will remain important for public health practitioners. This is especially true for practitioners who aspire to be, or who are in, leadership positions. Effective individual speakers retain their ability to target their messages precisely to meet the needs of particular audiences. Finally, the power of the spoken word provided to audiences through oral presentations will remain the major mode for persuasive communication.

CHAPTER 10 ENDNOTES

1. Bradt KM. *Story as a Way of Knowing.* Kansas City, MO: Sheed & Ward; 1997.
2. Crannell K. *Voice and Articulation.* Menlo Park, CA: Wadsworth, 2000.
3. Conference on Issues in Health Communication (sponsored by Annenberg School of Communication). June 6-8, 2000; New York, NY. CNN, June 6, 2000.
4. Schramm W. *The Process and Effects of Communication.* Urbana, IL: University of Illinois Press; 1954.
5. Berlo, D. *The Process of Communication.* New York: Holt, Reinhard and Winston; 1960.
6. Silvestri V. *Interpersonal Communication: Perspectives and Applications.* 3rd ed. Boston, MA: American Press; 1991.
7. Cooper L, ed. *The Rhetoric of Aristotle.* New York: Appleton-Century; 1932.
8. Morgan VM. Public speaking. In: Agricultural Communicators in Education *The Communicator's Handbook.* 3rd ed. Gainesville, FL: Maupin House; 1996.
9. McGinnis JM, Foege WH. Actual causes of death in the United States. *JAMA.*1993;270:2207-12.
10. Remington PL. Preventable causes of death in Wisconsin. *Wis Med J.* 1994;93:125-128.
11. Golden J. The persuasive power of ethos and image. In: Coleman WE, Berquist GF. Golden JL, eds: *Rhetoric of Western Thought.* 5th ed. Dubuque, IA: Kendall Hunt; 1995; 343-352.
12. Emerson EW, Forbes WE eds. *Journal of Ralph Waldo Emerson.* Boston: Houghton Miflin; 1912.
13. Andersen K, Clevenger T. Summary of experimental research on ethos. *Speech Monogr.* 29:59-73; 1963.
14. Grossberg L, et al. *Mediamaking: Mass Media in a Popular Culture.* Newbury Park, CA: Sage; 1998.
15. Weber, M. *Theory of social and economic organization.* New York: Oxford University Press; 1947.
16. Wallack L, Woodruff K, Dorfman L, Diaz I. *News for a Change: An Advocate's Guide to Working with the Media.* Thousand Oaks, CA: Sage; 1999.
17. Richards IA. *Philosophy of Rhetoric.* New York: Oxford; 1936.
18. Payne JG, Golden J. *Lectures in Professional Communication.* Boston, MA: Emerson College; 1991.
19. Coe N. A time to listen. *Am J Surgery.* 1997;173:534-537.
20. Levie WH, Lentz R. Effects of text illustrations: a review of research. *J Educational Psychol.* 1982;73:195-232.
21. Calvert P, ed. *The Communicator's Handbook: Tools, Techniques and Technology.* 4th ed. Gainesville, FL: Maupin House; 2000.
22. Markel M. *Technical Communication.* New York: Bedford/St. Martin's; 2000.
23. Centers for Disease Control and Prevention. *Scientific and Technical Information Simply Put: Tips for Creating Easy-To-Read Print Materials Your Audience Will Want to Read and Use.* 2nd ed. Atlanta, GA: Centers for Disease Control and Prevention, Office of Communication; 1999.

SUGGESTED READINGS AND RESOURCES

Calvert P, ed. *The Communicator's Handbook: Tools, Techniques and Technology.* 4th ed. Gainesville, FL: Maupin House; 2000.

Crannell K. *Voice and Articulation.* 4th ed. Menlo Park, CA: Wadsworth; 2000.

Ratzan SC, ed. Health Communication: Challenges for the 21st Century (Special Issue). *Am Behavior Scientist.* 1994;38:197-380.

Silvestri V. *Interpersonal Communication: Perspectives and Applications.* 3rd ed. Boston, MA: American Press; 1991.

The Patients' Network Web site. Available at http//www.iapo-pts.org.uk/tpn/tpn.html. Date of access: June 29, 2002.

Chapter Eleven

VISUAL COMMUNICATION

Isaac Lipkus, PhD
David E. Nelson, MD, MPH

Visual representation is an important vehicle for communicating health information. Despite its ubiquity, few public health professionals receive any training in visual communication, nor do they necessarily use the best approaches or recognize common problems. This chapter provides recommendations for using visuals to enhance the communication of information to nonscientific audiences.

BACKGROUND

Visual modalities are a common and popular means of communication. Although the full extent to which visual displays aid comprehension has yet to be rigorously researched, the impact of visuals should not be underestimated. There is evidence that visuals can enhance the interest of audiences and their retention of information.[1,2] This is not surprising, as humans are neurologically adapted to be highly receptive to visual images.[3]

Some forms of visual communication have a long history. The earliest graphs are believed to have been created in the 1300s, and Rene Descartes invented the modern 2-dimensional graph with x and y axes (Cartesian coordinates) in the early 17th century.[4] In the late 1700s and early 1800s, William Playfair developed line graphs, bar charts, and pie charts to display economic and demographic data.[5,6] Photography first began to develop in the 1830s.[7] Computer graphics have been a much more recent development.

Visual communication uses images, shapes, lines, diagrams, shading, pictures, and the layout of text to convey information. Graphs or charts (these words are used interchangeably in this chapter) are primarily used to illustrate statistics;[4] maps are used to illustrate geographic dispersion; and pictures are used to demonstrate important points, provide emotional context, or convey realism. Visual representation is often used as an adjunct to oral, written, and electronic communication,[3,8] and increasingly, audiences expect the use of visuals in communication activities.[9]

GENERAL CONSIDERATIONS

There are several general issues to consider when using visual communication. First, the visual item must attract the attention of the audience; if it is not noticed, it cannot convey information. Visuals should be relevant, esthetically pleasing, and delivered through a communication channel familiar to the intended audience. Second, they must enhance the presentation of information: visuals are rarely the primary means of communication; instead, they are usually used in conjunction with written, oral, and electronic communication.[1,8] The information in visuals should be integrated with these other forms of communication to enhance overall effectiveness. If not used in this manner, visuals will distract audiences from the main message.

Third, visuals should be relevant and tailored to the intended audience. There is increasing evidence on the effectiveness of tailoring messages to specific audiences by demographics or beliefs.[10] For example, subtle cues such as developing visuals that match the sex, race, or ethnicity characteristics of the audience, may enhance the likelihood that audiences will attend to the message. Fourth, visuals need to easily and accurately help audiences process, understand, retain, and use information. Keeping visuals simple for nonscientific audiences is a cardinal principle, and to maximize clarity, only one message per visual display should be generally be used.[11] Stressing certain features (highlighting key data points or text with color, large or bolded letters, or animation) makes an audience more likely to attend to the message.

PURPOSE, AUDIENCE, AND MESSAGE

As with other communication modalities, visuals are only a tool for conveying information. Public health practitioners must have a clear understanding of the purpose (why), audience (who), and the message (what) that they want to communicate before selecting a visual modality.

The initial concern in creating visual aids is the purpose, or why, of the communication activity. Is the main purpose of visual communication to provide information passively, assist audiences with informed decision-making, or persuade individuals or policymakers to make changes in behaviors, regulations, or laws? If the purpose is to persuade, it is especially critical to consider what form of visual communication will best capture the audience's attention.

As emphasized throughout this book, knowing the characteristics, beliefs, and needs of the audience is critical. The literacy and numeracy (understanding of mathematical concepts and numbers) of the target audience are especially critical for visual communication. Less literate and numerate individuals may have trouble with certain graphs and tables,[12,13] although the evidence of the effects of familiarity and experience of audiences with visual aids on how well people use and interpret information is not consistent.[14] Finally, it is necessary to decide on the main message to communicate to the audience, and the specific message that each visual is intended to convey,[14] for example, magnitude, comparisons, trends, geographic variation, sense of realism or emotion.[4,6,14-17]

SPECIFIC VISUAL COMMUNICATION MODALITIES

In public health, the most commonly used visual modalities are tables, line graphs, bar and pie charts, maps, pictures (drawings, photographs, clip art, diagrams, and videotape), and typography (text layout). The main features of each modality are summarized in Table 11.1.

TABLES

A table is the best choice when the goal is to stress a few specific pieces of information.[4,6] Primarily used for numbers, tables can also consist of symbols (apples to indicate daily servings of fruits, for instance) or a short list of related text items such as the major risk factors for low birth weight infants. Tables can be a viable option for displaying numbers when a large range exists between the highest and lowest numbers that may be difficult to convey in a graph.[4] A list of the actual causes of death in the United States is an appropriate use of a table (Table 11.2) because there is a large range in values from smoking (400,000 deaths) to illegal drug use (25,000 deaths).[18]

Tables should contain the minimum number of elements to communicate the main point, and they should contain few (if any) lines. Because tabular information must be decoded, tables are usually the least preferred visual communication modality to use with nonscientific audiences,[4] especially low-literacy and low-numeracy audiences. The key communication message should be immediately evident to audiences; unfortunately, tables often contain too many items (data overload) and do not rapidly convey a clear pattern.

BAR CHARTS

Bar charts, the most versatile means for displaying data visually, use either vertical or horizontal displays of bars or columns (Table 11.1). Histograms, paired bars, and stacked bar charts are common variations[4] (Figure 11.1). Bar charts are most often used to visually represent the magnitude of numbers and to compare groups, such as differences in diabetes prevalence by age group. Sometimes they are used to portray patterns over time,[4,19] but line graphs are the preferred means for displaying trends (see below). Stacked bar charts (Figure

TABLE 11.1 – SUMMARY OF MAJOR FORMS OF VISUAL COMMUNICATION IN PUBLIC HEALTH

Modality	Main Features	Major Uses
Table	Numbers in columns and rows	List specific numbers or text
Line Graph	Line(s) plotted on a grid over time	Examine trends
Bar Chart	Vertical or horizontal columns plotted on a grid	Highlight magnitude or comparison of numbers
Pie Chart	Divided circle that represents 100%	Display proportions totaling to 100%
Map	Geographic regions	Suggest geographic patterns or clusters
Picture	Actual or artistic representations of people, places, activities, or shapes	Demonstrate sequences of interrelated processes, enhance key features, evoke emotion, provide realism
Typography	Text	Highlight words through layout design

TABLE 11.2—SELECTED ACTUAL CAUSES OF DEATH IN THE UNITED STATES, 1990

Tobacco 400,000
Diet and physical activity 300,000
Alcohol 100,000
Firearms 35,000
Illicit use of drugs 20,000

Source: Adapted from Reference 18

11.1c) should be avoided, as decoding them is challenging.[15]

Bar charts will be most effective with nonscientific audiences if they contain only a few bars. For these audiences, a general rule is to include no more than six bars per graph. The following example from the National Cancer Institute demonstrates the versatility of bar charts.

BOX 11.1

The National Cancer Institute (NCI) was interested in developing comprehensible ways to communicate breast cancer risk.[20] The goals were to: (1) emphasize that breast cancer risk increases with age; and (2) encourage regular mammography screening among older women. After testing proposed materials with a focus group of women from the general public, NCI staff developed a visual display of bar charts showing in 10-year increments the number of women diagnosed nationally with breast cancer (Figure 11.2). Age groups with the most cases were highlighted in gray (women aged 40 years and older), and those with a lower incidence were left unshaded. NCI included the bar chart in breast cancer prevention materials.

LINE GRAPHS

Line graphs are very effective for displaying data over time, that is, trends[4] (Table 11.1). Time is generally plotted on the x-axis with the time units (years or months) equally spaced, the numbers to be graphed are plotted on the y-axis and the points on the graph connected by lines. Fundamentally, line graphs demonstrate whether numeric values are changing or staying the same over time. Variations include multiple lines, curvilinear approaches, and shaded graph areas underneath lines.[6,15] Line graphs can also be used to estimate the impact of programs, policies,[21] or perturbations at specific time periods[22] (Figure 11.3).

Line graphs can be effective with many nonscientific audiences. The biggest challenge for such graphs is avoiding the clutter of too many data lines (≤ 4 lines are recommended) or poor labeling.

PIE CHARTS

A pie chart is a divided circle used to represent visually proportions (percentages) that total 100%[4] (Table 11.1). They are sometimes displayed in three dimensions or with gaps between slices. Pie charts are especially good for highlighting either the largest or the smallest piece, e.g., that about half the population had four or more visits to health care providers in the past year[23] (Figure 11.4).

As a general rule, pie charts should use no more than six slices; the largest piece should be focused at "12 o'clock"; slices should be displayed clockwise in descending order; and labels should be short, horizontal, and outside of the pie.[4,8]

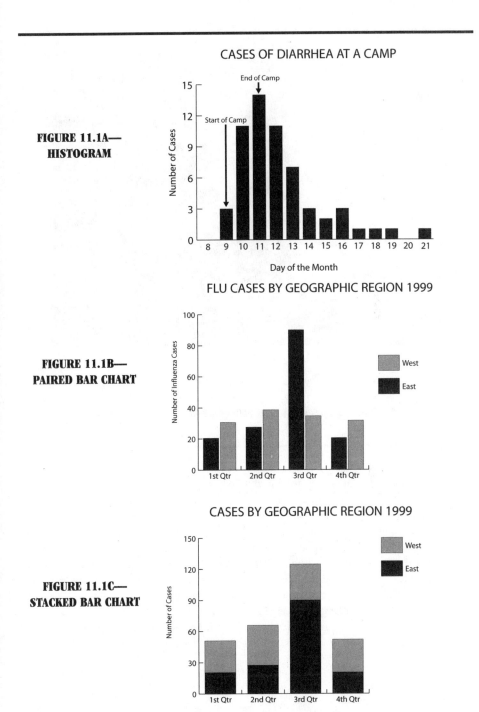

FIGURE 11.1A— HISTOGRAM

CASES OF DIARRHEA AT A CAMP

FIGURE 11.1B— PAIRED BAR CHART

FLU CASES BY GEOGRAPHIC REGION 1999

FIGURE 11.1C— STACKED BAR CHART

CASES BY GEOGRAPHIC REGION 1999

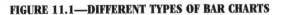

FIGURE 11.1—DIFFERENT TYPES OF BAR CHARTS

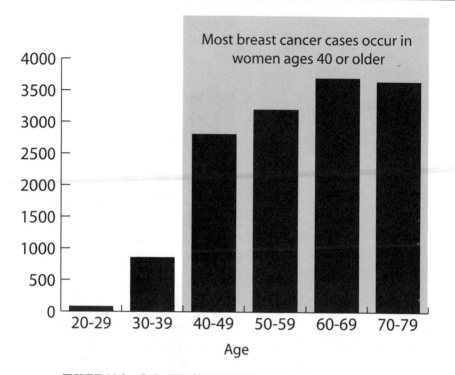

FIGURE 11.2—BAR CHART DEPICTING BREAST CANCER BY AGE

Source: Reference 20

MAPS

Mapping of data has long been used in public health practice to demonstrate geographic variation; John Snow's map of cholera cases in London is a legendary example.[6] Visually displaying data through maps remains a key activity for many public health practitioners. Advances in technology such as geocoding and the widespread availability of computer software (e.g., geographic information systems [GIS]), have made mapping a readily available format for communicating public health information. Mapping can be used to identify geographic clustering, and it can demonstrate local, county, state, or national variation in health measures, such as obesity[24] or mortality[25,26] (Figure 11.5). Shading and color in maps are important considerations (see below).

For most audiences, mapping is the best way to communicate geographic variability for public health data. As with line charts, it is essential to determine audience familiarity with maps and to minimize clutter.

PICTURES

Drawings, clip art, photographs, diagrams, and videotape are especially useful adjuncts to written, oral, and electronic communication, and they can also be used in conjunction

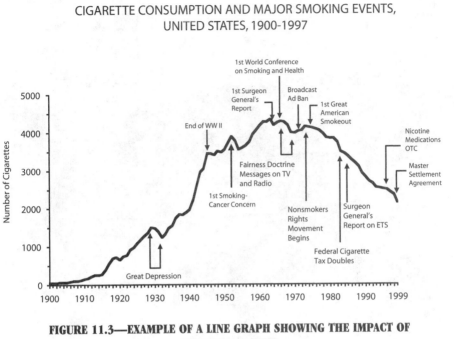

CIGARETTE CONSUMPTION AND MAJOR SMOKING EVENTS, UNITED STATES, 1900-1997

FIGURE 11.3—EXAMPLE OF A LINE GRAPH SHOWING THE IMPACT OF SELECTED EVENTS

Source: Adapted from Reference 22

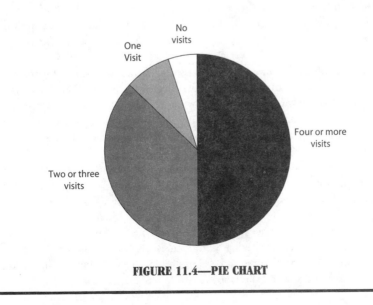

NUMBER OF VISITS TO A HEALTH PROFESSIONAL IN PAST YEAR

FIGURE 11.4—PIE CHART

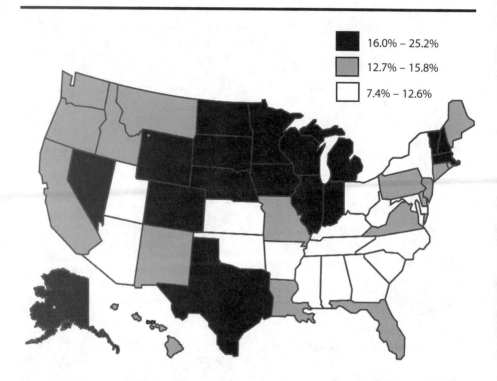

FIGURE 11.5—BINGE DRINKING BY STATE 1997-1999

with other forms of visual communication. Pictures are used to show sequences of interrelated processes, enhance key features (saliency), evoke emotions, and provide realism to communication activities[7,11,12] (Figure 11.6). Videos, because they include multiple pictures and sound, can also convey interactions between one or more parties and model activities or behaviors.

Pictures, unlike other visual modalities discussed so far, are well-suited for communicating non-quantitative information such as people affected by the issue being discussed, real-life events, nonverbal communication, and showing how causal events and processes unfold ("story lines").[11] Examples include photographs of injuries to children caused by land mines, diagrams demonstrating how nosocomial infections are spread in hospitals, and clip art (Figure 11.7).

Because most people are familiar with this mode of communication, pictures can be readily used with all nonscientific audiences. Although pictures can be used in multiple situations, they need to be tailored to enhance the goal and message of the communication activity. Pictures should not distract the audience from the intended messages(s) through extraneous factors meant to attract the target audience (i.e., making the picture too salient by dramatizing colors, unneeded background textures, etc.). Discussion and recommendations of the many forms of pictures and techniques for creating high-quality pictures for visual communication is beyond the scope of this book.

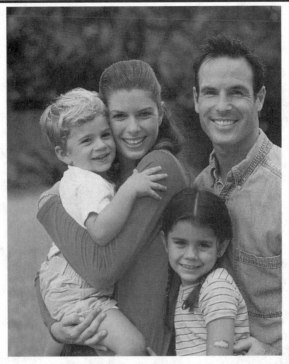

FIGURE 11.6—PHOTOGRAPH SUGGESTING FAMILY HAPPINESS

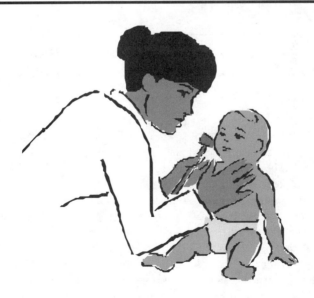

FIGURE 11.7—CLIP ART

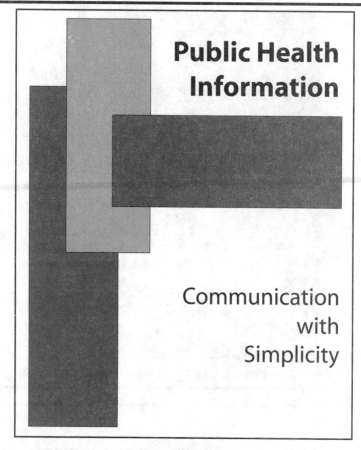

FIGURE 11.8—TYPOGRAPHIC LAYOUT FOR A REPORT

TYPOGRAPHY

The visual layout and display of text is the art of typography. In this chapter, the term will be used in the context of the visual layout of text for short written materials designed for the public (pamphlets or brochures) and for visuals used in oral presentations such as slides or overheads. The five important typographic considerations are proximity, alignment, repetition, contrast, and font (typeface) selection.[27]

Proximity means grouping common text elements close together; for example, Figure 11.8 groups the text together in the center of the page. Alignment is unifying every text object with the edge of some other text object; usually left or right alignments are preferred over centered alignments; (the text in Figure 11.8 is right aligned). Repetition is used to tie together separate parts of text design to create consistency; it can be created by using the same color, bullet, line, spacing, alignment, margins, bolding, font, clip art, etc. Repetition can be achieved for example, through the consistent use of the same font (typeface), or using the same logo, dividing line, etc. in the same location on each page.

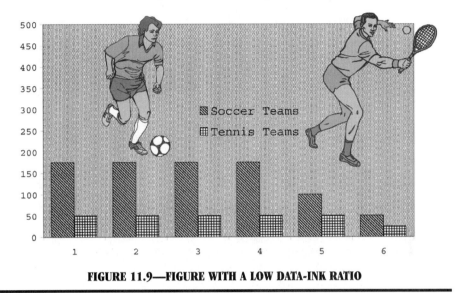

FIGURE 11.9—FIGURE WITH A LOW DATA-INK RATIO

Contrast, which is used to attract attention and to help organize the information, can be accomplished with lines, colors, fonts, or spatial relationships (different object sizes). To be effective, contrast must be strong; lack of contrast is why all capital letters should not be used to display text. Using different shadings for each rectangle creates contrast in Figure 11.8.

The four major categories of fonts are serif, sans serif, script, and ornate (serifs are the small strokes, or "feet," added to letters; sans serif is text without these strokes).[3,27] Serif fonts are best for written communications and sans serif fonts are best during oral presentations.[3,27] Script and ornate fonts are used to get attention but should be used sparingly, as they can distracting or difficult to read.

OTHER MODALITIES

Other visual displays less frequently used to present public health information to non-scientists include stick figures, box plots, scatter plots, risk ladders, Chernoff faces, dot charts, and volumetric displays. The reader is referred to reference 14 for a discussion of these modalities.

OTHER CONSIDERATIONS FOR VISUAL COMMUNICATION

DATA-INK RATIO

The data-ink ratio, which compares the amount of ink used for data with ink used for other aspects of the display should be as high as possible.[6] In practical terms, the designer should minimize extraneous lines, pictures, and other visual items that can distract readers from grasping the key points of a chart. Figure 11.9 is an example of a visual display with low data-ink ratio: the additional lines and objects distract and thus make it difficult to rapidly grasp key points. Horizontal and vertical lines on bar charts and line graphs should be avoided, as should shading or fill patterns on line graphs, as they lower the data-ink ratio and add clutter.[6]

COLOR AND SHADING

Color is an important component of visual design but should be considered carefully. For instance, if cost is a consideration or if materials are to be photocopied, black and white may be the best choice. If colors are to be added, they should be used sparingly, and usually no more than two or three different colors should be used. When more than one visual is required, the same colors should be used consistently.

For color combinations, the key principle is to use colors with strong contrast.[8] Light green, yellow, orange, and red are considered warm colors, while dark green, blue, and purple are considered cool colors. Warm colors tend to "jump out" at audiences, while cool colors tend to recede. Because of these characteristics, the most effective combination is warm-colored objects set against cool-colored backgrounds. Colors that are complementary opposites of each other–blue and orange, red and green–should not be used together, as they tend to compete for attention. Table 11.3 lists the recommended color combinations to use and those to avoid.

In different cultures, some colors convey specific meanings. In the U.S., red typically communicates threat, anger, fire, or warning (for example, a stop sign or a thermometer); blue conveys cold, cool, or water; green communicates nature or money; yellow conveys caution.[8] However, attention to cultural meaning is important when considering using color to convey a particular meaning; for example, red signals happiness in China. Because most audiences have expectations about the meaning of certain colors, practitioners are best served by following color conventions. For example, red is usually a good choice for indicating high risk and blue a good choice for low risk in the United States.

Shading (hues) of individual colors, including black and gray, can also graphically convey information, especially in maps.[14] Making a single color darker can represent significantly higher risks, rates, or numbers. Shading on maps often reveals geographic patterns or clusters.[14] When shading is used, color choice must be carefully considered, the shading pattern must be consistent if used on more than one visual, and generally no more than three distinct colors should be used.

Color is not always the best choice for visually communicating public health information through tables and charts,[8] since it can draw viewers' attention away from key infor-

TABLE 11.3—RECOMMENDED COLOR COMBINATIONS TO USE AND THOSE TO AVOID

Recommended color combinations:
Black and white
Black and yellow
Blue and yellow
Blue and white

Color combinations to avoid:
Red and green
Blue and red
White and yellow
Light green and yellow
Gray and yellow

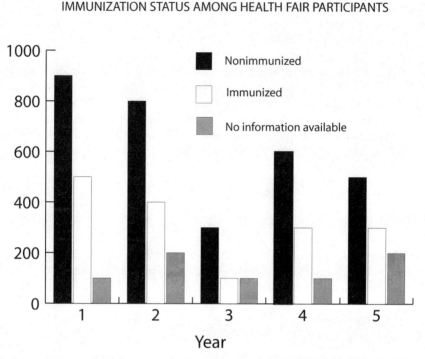

IMMUNIZATION STATUS AMONG HEALTH FAIR PARTICIPANTS

FIGURE 11.10—PAIRED BAR CHART WITH FILL PATTERNS THAT MAXIMIZE CONTRAST

mation elements.[6] For example, if color photographs or pictures are part of the visual communication activity, black-and-white figures or charts may be better choices.

FILL PATTERNS

Fill patterns are the ink styles (usually black or gray) used on bars, pie slices, or geographic areas (maps).[4] (As mentioned in a previous section, because of low data-ink ratio, using fill patterns on line graphs is not recommended.) Examples of fill patterns include solid color, outline with a clear interior, vertical lines, horizontal lines, diagonal lines, and cross-hatched lines. When using these patterns, it is essential to minimize the use of ink and to select patterns that maximize contrast. For nonscientific audiences, generally no more than three fill patterns should be used[4] (Figure 11.10).

TITLES, LABELS, AND LEGENDS

To maximize utility, a title should be short and easily distinguished from the rest of the graphic (perhaps through the use of larger fonts or boldface type), and it should emphasize the key communication point. For example, a title such as "Smoking Increases the Risk of Cervical Cancer" on a bar chart that compares the relative risk of this disease for smokers and nonsmokers would stress the important communication message.

Labels, which are written text used directly on visual displays for descriptive purposes, should be simple and short. They include text within the body of a chart or graph, such as y- and x-axis descriptors, as well as text that highlights a key data feature within the body of the chart or graph. Labels for time elements (e.g., years) on line graphs can be especially problematic if data are available for multiple time periods. One solution is to use labels for certain years (e.g., 1985, 1990, 1995) and tick marks for the other years. Labels are also used to highlight key data points. For example, bolded or enlarged text on a bar chart can stress a maximum allowable exposure limit to an environmental or occupational chemical. For a line graph, including text with an arrow can highlight high or low values attributable to specific events, such as a policy change, outbreak, or a war (Figure 11.3).

Legends are the text (or often numeric values for maps) that describes what the lines, bars, pie slices, shading, or fill patterns represent, such as men vs. women; high, medium, or low. For nonscientific audiences, legends should be placed directly on or near the appropriate line, bar, or pie slice rather than in a separate location such as a box.

CHALLENGES AND BARRIERS

CLUTTER

Visual clutter, or chart junk, results from trying to cram too much information into tables or charts and obscures the main points to be communicated.[6] Examples include using too much text or too many numbers, lines, bars, pie slices, pictures, colors, or patterns. A good example of excess complexity is a line chart with two or more lines with different y-axis values and legends. While perhaps appropriate for a scientific audience, it is unlikely to be readily understood by nonscientists. One message per visual display is a good rule for minimizing complexity and clutter.[11]

EXCESSIVE USE OF VISUALS

Using too many visuals is another common problem. Because of their backgrounds and interests, some practitioners overuse visuals to make their points. Instead of using one simple visual display to make a key point (or sometimes even just a few words), multiple graphs and pictures are used, thereby defeating the goal of making the communication activity simple and easily understood. When it is necessary to use multiple graphs (for example, to show how several risks factors affect a common outcome), legends, labels, scales, and colors should be consistent to allow smooth transitions across graphs.[14]

DISTRACTION

Visual distractions are the use of tangential communication techniques or approaches to increase audience attention ("bells and whistles"). With the availability of sophisticated software packages, color graphics, digital photography, and videos, it is now fairly easy to create multimedia extravaganzas. In an oral presentation, for example, it is probably not necessary to have text or numbers arrive from the left, right, top, or bottom, or to add extra sounds.

Although fancy visual presentations may be the norm in occupations such as sales, in public health they may be distracting and perceived by some audiences as an attempt to "sell" them something, which may reduce the speaker's credibility. Careful knowledge of audiences and their expectations is essential when deciding how many audiovisual "extras" to include in presentations.

DISTORTION

Another frequent problem is spatial distortion. The most common example is adjusting the interval width on the y- or x-axis on line or bar charts to maximize or minimize differences between groups or to maximize or minimize trends.[4,6,28,29] Figures 11.11a and 11.11b show the same data on the prevalence of per capita alcohol consumption from 1977 to 1996[30] but with different y-axis interval widths. An audience's perception of this information would likely differ, depending on which figure was used. Trend data can also be subject to misuse or distortion by changing the x-axis to show different starting or ending dates or by modifying interval widths. The use of tick marks on y- and x-axes is one way to reduce biases in perceptions, as are reference points (a bolded number on the y-axis or symbols such as arrows to indicate higher risk).

Volume distortion can be another problem.[8] Human or other figures are sometimes used to depict quantities or relative differences. But because individuals demonstrate important biases when estimating physical magnitudes of visual objects,[4,6] such figures should not be used to represent quantities or differences. Other than volume distortion for quantities or differences, no one rule for distortion applies to all situations. Sometimes a small change is important and needs to be highlighted: a one percentage point increase in the prevalence of diabetes is enormous when compared with a one percentage point increase in the prevalence of adult women who received a pap test in the past 3 years.

Being accurate is the key to avoiding distortion and misuse.[6] Many software programs use an automatic scaling feature for graphs that may or may not be appropriate for data to be presented; this can be especially problematic when using multiple graphs.

THREE-DIMENSIONAL DISPLAYS

Three-dimensional graphical displays are sometimes used with bar and pie charts, but should be avoided. Although they can make individual bar and pie slices stand out, all the bars or pie slices become more noticeable,[3] thus diminishing the desired effect. Furthermore, such images reduce data-ink ratio without adding additional information.

STATISTICAL UNCERTAINTY

Trying to explain statistical uncertainty to nonscientific audiences is challenging, and few visuals are known to be effective at communicating uncertainty.[14] This is not surprising, given that displaying statistical uncertainty requires higher levels of numeracy and decoding skills. Box plots may work with some audiences, but other visual communication forms common to the scientific community, such as scatter plots or 95% confidence interval bars, should be avoided with nonscientists.

SUMMARY

Visual displays are commonly used in conjunction with oral, written, and electronic communication to enhance the understanding, use, and retention of information. Visuals should attract audience attention, enhance information presentation, be tailored to the audience, and communicate information easily and accurately. The familiarity of audiences with the type of visual modality, as well as the audience's literacy and numeracy, are important considerations.

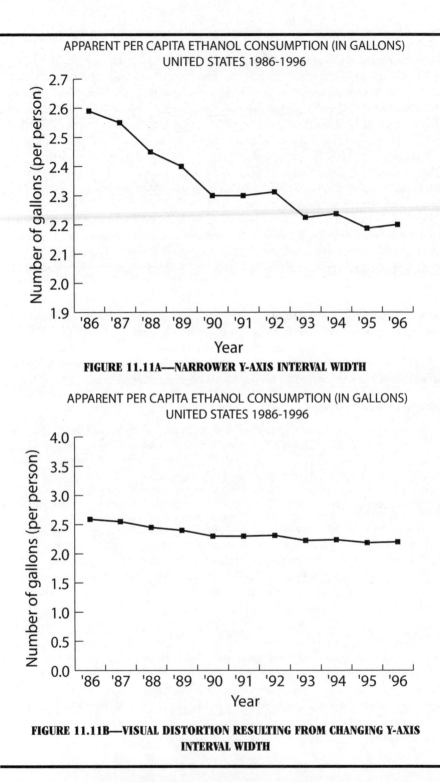

APPARENT PER CAPITA ETHANOL CONSUMPTION (IN GALLONS)
UNITED STATES 1986-1996

FIGURE 11.11A—NARROWER Y-AXIS INTERVAL WIDTH

APPARENT PER CAPITA ETHANOL CONSUMPTION (IN GALLONS)
UNITED STATES 1986-1996

FIGURE 11.11B—VISUAL DISTORTION RESULTING FROM CHANGING Y-AXIS
INTERVAL WIDTH

Various modalities are best suited for different purposes: tables for displaying a few elements; line graphs for trends; bar charts for magnitude or relative differences; pie charts for proportions; maps for geographic differences; and pictures for evoking emotion and showing a sequences of interrelated processes. Additional issues to consider include data-ink ratio, color, shading, fill patterns, labeling, and legends. Common problems include clutter, use of too many visuals, distraction, distortion, three-dimensional displays, and uncertainty.

The importance of visual displays as a means of communicating public health information is likely to increase, given the continued advances in technology. Use of the Internet is likely to expand, and visual communication plays a key role in this type of communication. There are now several powerful and widely available graphics/graphic presentation software packages (e.g., Powerpoint, Corel Draw) that allow practitioners to create effective visuals easily. Digital photography and scanning technology can be used to include photographs, clip art, and diagrams with oral, written, and electronic communication materials.

Given the daily visual bombardment experienced by most Americans, there is a growing need for practitioners to understand how to create and present visual health information to positively influence the public's health. Fortunately, the growing sophistication of electronic software and hardware should make it easier to create visual displays tailored to specific audiences. Such techniques may increase the likelihood that the information is read, retained, and used. Finally, because of its potential to communicate information rapidly and effectively, visual communication will likely play an increasing role in trying to reduce information overload by helping audiences focus on key points.

CHAPTER 11 ENDNOTES

1. Calvert P, ed. *The Communicator's Handbook: Tools, Techniques and Technology.* 4th ed. Gainesville, FL: Maupin House; 2000.
2. Levie WH, Lentz R. Effects of text illustrations: a review of research. *J Educ Psychol.* 1982;73:195-232.
3. Gatlin PL. Visuals and prose in manuals: the effective combination. In: *Proceedings of the 35th International Technical Communication Conference*, Arlington, VA; 1988: 113-115.
4. Holmes N. *Designer's Guide to Creating Charts and Diagrams.* New York: Watson-Guptill; 1991.
5. Playfair W. *The Commercial and Political Atlas.* London, England: Debrett; 1787.
6. Tufte ER. *The Visual Display of Quantitative Information.* Cheshire, CT: Graphics Press; 1983.
7. McDarrah FW, McDarrah GS. *The Photography Encyclopedia.* New York: Schirmer; 1999.
8. Markel M. *Technical Communication.* 6th ed. New York: Bedford/St. Martins; 2000.
9. Brockmann RJ. *Writing Better Computer Use Documentation: From Paper to Hypertext.* New York: Wiley; 1990.
10. Skinner CB, Campbell MK, Rimer BK, Curry S, Prochaska JO. How effective is tailored print communication? *Ann Behavioral Med.* 1999; 21: 290-298.
11. Centers for Disease Control and Prevention, Office of Communication. *Scientific and Technical Information Simply Put: Tips for Creating Easy-To-Read Print Materials Your Audience Will Want to Read and Use*, 2nd ed. Atlanta, GA: Centers for Disease Control and Prevention, Office of Communication; 1999.
12. Root J, Stableford S. *Write It Easy-to-Read: A Guide to Creating Plain English Materials.* Biddeford ME: Maine AHEC Health Literacy Center; 1997.
13. Lipkus IM, Samsa G, Rimer BK. General performance on a numeracy scale among highly educated samples. *Med Decis Making.* 2001;21:37-44.
14. Lipkus I, Hollands JG. The Visual Communication of Risk. *Monogr Natl Cancer Inst.* 1999;25:149-163.
15. Cleveland WS, McGill R. Graphical perception: Theory, experimentation, and application to the development of graphic methods. *J Am Stat Assoc.* 1984; 70:531-554.

16. Johnson BB, Slovic P. Presenting uncertainty in health risk assessment: initial studies of its effects on risk perception and trust. *Risk Anal* 1995; 15: 485-494.

17. Kaplan RM, Hammel B, Schimmel LE. Patient information processing and decision to accept treatment. *J Soc Behav Pers.* 1985; 1: 113-120.

18. McGinnis JM, Foege WH. Actual causes of death in the United States. *JAMA.* 1993;270:2207-12.

19. Davis K. Medicaid: *The Health Care Safety Net for the Nation's Poor.* Testimony before the Committee on Finance, The United States Senate, Hearing on Welfare and Medicaid Reform, June 19, 1996. New York: The Commonwealth Fund.

20. National Cancer Institute. *How the Public Perceives, Processes and Interprets Risk Information: Findings from Focus Group Research with the General Public.* Bethesda, MD: National Cancer Institute; 1998: Report No. POS-T086.

21. Nelson DE, Bolen J, Kresnow M. Trends in safety belt use by demographics and by type of state safety belt law, 1987-1993. *Am J Public Health.* 1998;88:245-249.

22. Giovino GA, Schooley MW, Zhu BP, Chrismon JH, Tomar SL, Peddicord JP, Merritt RK, Husten CG, Eriksen MP. Surveillance for selected tobacco-use behaviors—United States, 1990-1994. *MMWR CDC Surv Summ.* 1994;43:1-43.

23. National Center for Health Statistics. *Health, United States, 2001 With Urban and Rural Health Chartbook.* Hyattsville, Maryland: 2001.

24. Mokdad AH, Serdula MK, Dietz WH, Bowman BA, Marks JS, Koplan JP. The spread of the obesity epidemic in the United States, 1991-1998. *JAMA.* 1999;282:1519-1522.

25. Pickle LW, Mungiole M, Jones GK, White AA. *Atlas of United States Mortality.* Hyattsville, MD: Centers for Disease Control and Prevention, National Center for Health Statistics; 1996; DHHS Publication No. (PHS) 97-1015.

26. National Cancer Institute. Surveillance, Epidemiology, and End Results. Available at http://seer.cancer.gov. Date accessed: June 22, 2002.

27. Williams R. *The Non-Designers Design Book: Design and Typographic Principles for the Visual Novice.* Berkeley, CA: Peachpit Press, 1994.

28. Huff D, Geiss I. *How to Lie with Statistics.* New York: WW Norton & Company; 1993.

29. Spirer HF, Spirer L, Jaffe AJ. *Misused Statistics,* 2nd ed. New York: Marcel Dekker; 1998.

30. Williams GD, Stinson FS, Sanchez LL, Dufour MC. *Apparent Per Capita Alcohol Consumption: National, State, and Regional Trends.* Bethesda, MD: National Institute on Alcohol Abuse and Alcoholism; 1998: Surveillance Report #47.

SUGGESTED READINGS AND RESOURCES

Lipkus IM, Hollands JG. The visual communication of risk. *Monogr Natl Cancer Inst.* 1999;25:149-163.

Markel M. *Technical Communication.* 6th ed. New York: Bedford/St. Martin's Press; 2000.

Pickle LW, Mungiole M, Jones GK, White AA. *Atlas of United States Mortality.* Hyattsville, MD: Centers for Disease Control and Prevention, National Center for Health Statistics; 1996: DHHS Publication No. (PHS) 97-1015.

Tufte ER. *The Visual Display of Quantitative Information.* Cheshire, CT: Graphics Press; 1983.

Williams R. *The Non-Designers Design Book: Design and Typographic Principles for the Visual Novice.* Berkeley, CA: Peachpit Press; 1994.

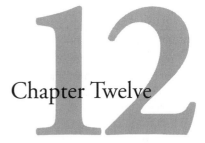

Chapter Twelve

ELECTRONIC COMMUNICATION

Scott C. Ratzan MD, MPA, MA
David E. Nelson, MD, MPH
Thomas R. Eng, VMD, MPH
Carmelle Goldberg, MSc

dvances in information and communication technology provide new opportunities to communicate about public health. Electronic mail (e-mail), Web sites, interactive TV, and instant messaging are examples of new communication media that provide unprecedented global access to people and information on a scale unimaginable 10 years ago. This chapter provides a brief overview of electronic communication and applications commonly used in public health practice.

BACKGROUND

Electronic communication may represent the most substantial change in communication since the invention of the printing press. The Internet, in particular, has catalyzed a dramatic evolution in distance-based education, marketing, finance and commerce, information access, and entertainment. The application of emerging information and communication to health issues is evolving at a somewhat slower pace than other sectors of the economy, but may still spur innovative solutions for longstanding problems in health and health care, such as quality, access, and cost.[1] Nevertheless, the Internet has greatly expanded the access of consumers to unprecedented amounts of health information through health-related Web sites, e-mail, listservs, and electronic bulletin boards.

Electronic communication is not a distinct form of communication but a medium for transmitting written, audio, and visual information. A strict definition is difficult because of the rapidly evolving and converging technologies. The term *electronic communication* in this chapter refers to the use of a computer or other electronic device (e.g., Internet appliance, interactive television, personal communicator) to access or exchange information among individuals.[2-4] Detailed descriptions of all forms of electronic communication are beyond the scope of this book; instead, this chapter focuses on e-mail and Web sites, as these are already widely used in public health practice.

E-mail connects millions of individuals worldwide and is the most popular Internet application. Of the more than 140 million Internet users in the United States, more than 80% use e-mail.[5] With a wide range of uses, it has become the dominant means of communication in many organizations. The primary means of e-mail communication is text-based, although technological advances allow for multimedia messages. Adjuncts to e-mail include listservs, which are e-mail user groups of persons interested in specific topics, and electronic bulletin boards, which provide users with a public area for posting and reviewing electronic messages.

The Internet links distant and disparate computers and computer systems worldwide through a standard communications protocol. The World Wide Web ("the Web"), which depends on the Internet to function, is a distributed network of information based on a standard communication protocol (hypertext markup language [HTML]) and format for describing the structure of documents. A Web site location or address (uniform resource locator [URL]) on the Internet contains written, visual, or audio information developed by the sponsor. Sites are hosted on computer servers and accessed through a graphical interface called a Web browser.

Electronic communication has several general features that differentiate it from other modes of communication (Table 12.1). The benefits of electronic communication include interactivity; capacity to transmit information through multiple methods (written, visual, or audio); rapid transmission of information; potential to reach large audiences; ability to transcend geographic and political boundaries; creation of new communication networks among people with similar interests or experiences; individualized (tailored) messages; mode of delivery; asynchronicity (individuals can use it any time of day or night); and reduction of communication costs (e.g., long distance phone bills, printing, or mailing expenses).[3,6,7]

TABLE 12.1—BENEFITS AND CHALLENGES OF ELECTRONIC COMMUNICATION

Benefits:
  Interactivity
  Multiple methods for communication (written, visual, audio)
  Rapid transmission of information
  Reaches large number of individuals
  Transcends geographic and political boundaries
  Creates networks of people
  Individualized (tailored) communication
  Asynchronous (information accessed when user wishes to)
  Reduces cost of communication

Challenges:
  Accessibility (gap between those with and without access to information technology)
  Literacy problems for some users (reading level, ability to use computers)
  Rapidly changing hardware and software
  Lack of privacy and confidentiality
  E-mail overload
  Locating appropriate Web sites
  Highly variable quality of information
  Assurance of information security (e.g., viruses, network intrusion)
  Maintenance (changing e-mail and Web site addresses, blind links)

GENERAL CONSIDERATIONS FOR ELECTRONIC COMMUNICATION IN PUBLIC HEALTH

Its global reach, interactivity, and ability to provide large quantities of information make electronic communication an important tool for public health practitioners. Table 12.2 lists specific current and potential uses for this means of public health communication.

The practice of public health relies heavily on the ongoing collection, analysis, and dissemination of information.[8] Electronic communication can provide a means to collect data and other information rapidly for public health surveillance and monitoring of community health indicators. In the future, "disease surveillance" may be blended into a larger system of "health surveillance," and a substantial proportion of health information and data may be generated by the routine collection of data from many community settings rather than from reports of clinical encounters. The National Electronic Disease Surveillance System (NEDSS)[9] is likely to develop more quickly because of the advances in electronic communication that may lead to both more accurate community health monitoring and improved detection of disease outbreaks.[10]

Electronic communication can be used as a means to collect survey data. Internet-based surveys, using samples based on e-mail addresses, are already widely used to obtain data from certain populations such as professional groups. Panel surveys of individuals based on using e-mail lists as sampling frames are now being conducted.[11] Internet-based surveys of the general population in public health are not widespread, however, because of concerns about the representativeness of sampled populations. As more individuals have Internet access, however, and as response rates to other survey modes continue to decline, use of Internet-based surveys is likely to increase.

Internet surveys offer potential advantages over other survey modes. These include lower

TABLE 12.2—CURRENT AND POTENTIAL USES OF ELECTRONIC COMMUNICATION IN PUBLIC HEALTH

Information Collection
Surveillance
Surveys
Evaluation

Information and Training Provision
Locating information
Disseminating information
Distance-based learning

Networking
To other health professionals
Among nonscientific audiences (e.g., groups for support, guidance, and information-sharing)

Interventions
Tailored health communication
Advocacy

Other Uses
Telemedicine
Clinical information systems

cost, easier sample selection, completion at respondents' convenience, easy ability to provide incentives, ability to use visual aids and audio to enhance survey attractiveness, rapid follow-up with nonrespondents, tailoring of questions to specific audiences, ability to reduce data collection and input errors, ease of data collection and data processing, and rapid data analysis. Internet-based surveys also have challenges that go beyond the representativeness of sampled populations, however, such as the need to develop effective design layouts and the tendency of users to skim Internet text.[12,13] The quality of data from Internet-based surveys compared with telephone or household interview surveys is unclear.

Another public health use of electronic communication is evaluation, especially formative and process evaluation.[14] Because of the ease of selecting potential respondents (including those with certain demographic characteristics), the ability to use audio, written, and video communication, and the ability to access the medium at a time that is convenient for the user, electronic communication provides an inexpensive and rapid means to pre-test materials with both professional and nonprofessional audiences through focus groups. It can also be used for other types of qualitative research. Because of the ease of tracking (for example, determining the number of visitors to a Web site or the number of e-mails) and ability to profile users, electronic communication can provide a means to conduct process evaluation and estimate whether communication messages are actually being delivered to intended audiences.

One of the most important functions of public health practitioners, especially those employed by government agencies or private health organizations, is to disseminate information to multiple audiences.[15] Electronic communication has revolutionized information dissemination. Large numbers of publications, data sets, and conference presentations can now be made available through the Internet. Material previously available only through libraries can be obtained from Web sites, and scientific literature searches can be done rapidly, often at no cost (chapter 3).[16] Information materials can be targeted to selected audiences such as journalists, health professionals, or the general public,[17,18] and the need to produce hard copy publications (and their attendant costs) has been substantially reduced. Electronic communication can also improve the reach and use of public health services by increasing awareness of available services and expanding community outreach, especially to rural areas where distance has been a significant barrier to service delivery.

In addition to disseminating information to other audiences, public health practitioners are also consumers of public health information, and Web sites can be an excellent resource. The Internet is especially valuable for locating the "gray literature;" that is, information on less popular or rare topics that is often difficult to find. The Internet is commonly used for training, such as on-line courses or seminars. For many public health disciplines, Internet-based training is likely to become more important over time. Reasons for this include time and resource constraints for travel, lower cost, availability of on-line support, and the opportunity for more one-on-one interaction with instructors and other students.

Networking is among the most important uses of electronic communication for public health practitioners. It provides a means to communicate interactively with professional and nonprofessional audiences on an unprecedented scale, as experiences, approaches, recommendations, and data can be rapidly and widely communicated with multiple audiences. Networking can be used for many purposes in public health, from creating support groups of persons trying to quit smoking to "action alert" networks for advocacy purposes.

Electronic communication can also be used for public health interventions to persuade audiences through health education, social marketing, or advocacy. Because of the capacity to segment audiences, electronic communication can be used to develop health education and behavioral change materials for specific populations (smokers or diabetics, for example). Tailored health communication using electronic means has been shown to be effective in some populations,[19,20] although research has been limited and primarily focused on informed decision-making and behavior change among individuals in the general public.[21, 22] Electronic communication interventions, however, are also possible with other public health audiences, such as the news media, private health organizations, and advocacy groups.

Finally, electronic communication can be used to enhance patient care and health care practice management through telemedicine (the online delivery of healthcare services and electronic transmission of clinical information such as radiographs and laboratory tests), and clinical information systems such as electronic medical records, financial systems, or tracking systems.[1]

PURPOSE, AUDIENCE, AND MESSAGE

As with other forms of communication, practitioners must first consider the purpose, audience, and message(s) for electronic communication. It is important to recognize that e-mail is a passive means of communication, and receivers have great leeway in reading or responding to messages. Practitioners should consider whether using the Web is the best choice for information retrieval. The Web can be a powerful way to locate recent public health information from a variety of sources; however, if the same information is readily available in published forms such as reference books, textbooks and reports, searching the Web may be time consuming and frustrating. When providing information on Web sites for others, clarifying the purpose is equally important, as it guides the design of the site and decisions about which materials to make available.

Directly related to the purpose for electronic communication is to know the audience and their preferred communication channels. The use and acceptability of electronic communication varies widely among nonscientific audiences. In general, younger persons are embracing computers and the Internet more avidly than are persons in other age groups.[21] Regardless of age, some members of the general population have low computer and reading literacy skills and have difficulty understanding how to use e-mail and "surf" the web.[21] Before using e-mail or posting materials on a Web site, practitioners should consider whether their target audience might prefer another means of communication. There are many situations for which a phone call, letter, or a face-to-face meeting is more appropriate than electronic communication. For example, although most people in private health organizations and the news media are comfortable using electronic media, e-mail or Web sites may not be the best choice for reaching certain administrators and other people with tight and frequently changing time schedules.

It is necessary to consider the message (what) to communicate. This is usually straightforward in e-mails for interpersonal use; however, when e-mail is used to reach nonscientific audiences, it is important to consider the main communication message. Similarly, deciding what to communicate is also necessary with Web sites: what materials are the most appropriate to communicate the intended messages on Web sites? Finally, there are ethical considerations with electronic, as with other forms, of communication, that practitioners need to consider. Questions to ask include: Should proactive communication "push" certain information on audiences selectively? Will the communication "do good" or at the least "do no harm"? Will the audience be able to decipher and decide the appropriate use of information for ideal health?

SPECIFIC RECOMMENDATIONS FOR E-MAIL

Because of its widespread availability and the different uses and approaches for reaching audiences via e-mail (messages to friends, reports to colleagues, messages to elected officials for advocacy purposes), this section will focus on recommendations applicable for most situations.[23]

The familiarity and use of e-mail by people varies greatly: some find it a novelty, while others are overloaded with e-mail messages and often ignore them. Because it can be used to send and receive messages rapidly, simple e-mail messages often substitute for telephone conversations or face-to-face meetings. E-mail should be used with some caution—users should be bear in mind that their work-site electronic messages can usually be traced and restored even after being deleted, and unintended people may read non-encrypted messages. As a general rule, it is best not to put anything in an e-mail that the sender would not write on a postcard or see as a newspaper headline.

Table 12.3 lists recommendations for composing and responding to e-mail messages. Practitioners need to be especially wary of sending or responding to controversial e-mails and consider how each message they send would be perceived if it were to be widely distributed. If a controversial message is received, it is better to discuss the issues or concerns with the sender face-to-face or by telephone.

SPECIFIC RECOMMENDATIONS FOR WEB SITES

Given the plethora of health-related Web sites, finding appropriate sites and determining the quality of information they provide are becoming important issues for public health practitioners. Understanding the principles of Web site design can help practitioners who have input into the design or the materials to be placed on Web sites.

FINDING WEB SITES

Locating useful Web sites for all topics, including public health, is a challenge. Table 3.5 and appendices 1 and 2 list selected Web sites for locating public health information, but these sites will not meet the needs of all practitioners. Web site directories, search engines, meta-search engines, and meta-crawlers can help users narrow the list of available sites.

TABLE 12.3—GENERAL GUIDELINES FOR USE OF E-MAIL IN PUBLIC HEALTH PRACTICE

Use subject line
Send messages only to the appropriate people
Keep messages short
Do not use all capital letters
Do not include sensitive or personal information (how it would read as a newspaper headline?)
Think carefully before responding to controversial e-mails
Avoid sending or forwarding emotional, inspirational, or humorous messages
Use reminder messages, but do so sparingly

Directories and search engines act as indexes: users type in the key word or phrase, and receive a list of Web sites that contain that word or phrase. Some search engines can also be used to locate specific graphic or audio files. Commonly used general directories, search engines, and meta-search engines are described in references 24, 25, and 26. In addition, there are search engines that specialize in specific topical searches such as finding medical-related sites.[27]

Regardless of the type of search engine, it is essential to use the most specific or descriptive word or phrase possible. Use of a general term such as "cancer," for example, may return millions of "hits" for this word from Web sites.[28] Note, however, that the Internet has grown so large that the best search engines can catalogue only a small percentage of the information available on the World Wide Web.[29]

QUALITY OF INFORMATION ON WEB SITES

The quality of information on Web sites is a major concern. Web sites, listserves, and electronic bulletin boards are essentially unregulated, thus the information they provide can range from the state-of-the-art consensus to complete hogwash. There are many published criteria for evaluating the quality of health-related information available on the Internet (e.g., references 2, 30, and 31). Some general principles can help practitioners locate higher quality Web sites. These principles are relevant not only for evaluating the Web sites of others, but also for assessing Web sites sponsored by practitioners' own work organizations. Web site quality issues cover both the sponsor (who) and the content (what). Some information about the quality of a Web site can be assessed by evaluating the sponsor, and sites should clearly state their sponsor. Is the sponsor's name recognizable, and is it a well-recognized entity with a good reputation? The extension of the Web site address usually indicates whether the sponsor is a commercial firm (.com or .biz), a government agency (.gov), an organization (.org), or an educational institution (.edu), whereas a ".net", ".us", or ".info" extension is a heterogeneous designation.

Knowing who sponsors a site can provide insight into its purpose. Practitioners should recognize that the underlying reason for making information available on-line can be affected by conflicts of interest. These conflicts may be rooted in commerce (selling products or advertising) or by supporting a particular policy or viewpoint. Finally, as an ethical responsibility, sponsors of Web sites should notify users whether user confidentiality and anonymity are protected and if not, who will have access to user information.[21]

The content of information on Web sites is, not surprisingly, closely related to the sponsor. Does the information provided include appropriate documentation, such as citations of authors or references to well-established journals or reports? Is the information current, scientifically credible, and coherent with the existing body of scientific evidence? Information should be suspect if it is based primarily on testimonials, secrets, or new findings; if it is based on statements from persons with unknown or questionable credentials; if it contradicts the bulk of prior research, is not dated, or has not been reviewed by other scientists; or if it attempts to sell unproven products.[32] Content issues are especially relevant for practitioners who place their materials on their own work organizations' Web sites. Information should not be placed on Web sites unless it has undergone the same scrutiny that print documents would receive, which includes the careful checking of data or other information, limitations, and citations when appropriate.

SPECIFIC RECOMMENDATIONS FOR WEB SITE DESIGN

The last consideration is the quality of the Web site design. Few practitioners are Web designers, yet familiarity with basic principles is important, as many public health professionals have input into the design and content of Web sites. Poor Web design will discourage people from accessing, let alone using, information.[12]

Because one design does not work for all audiences, tailoring of materials is necessary; if one goal of the site is to reach the general public, materials developed specifically for scientists or the news media are not likely to be appropriate. Fortunately, through recent Web site development techniques, materials can be tailored fairly easily to different audiences. A team approach should be used to ensure that public health subject matter experts, Web designers, and when possible, representatives of the intended audiences, have an opportunity to contribute to the Web site design layout and the materials to be made available. Such an approach will help avoid the common problem of poorly designed sites.

Recommendations on Web site design are listed in Table 12.4. Web site design needs to be consistent, and whenever possible, include the sponsor's name (and logo, if applicable), the same color scheme, and layout on each page. Using specific layout designs and navigation approaches are key components of successful sites. Layout must capture the attention of users and provide them with easy-to-find information. A technique commonly used to create "user-friendly" Web pages is to start each hypertext page with a short conclusion; this is known as the inverse pyramid approach and is often used by newspaper reporters. Providing detailed background information on a given topic, especially at the beginning of a page, should be avoided, as only a small number of users will want detailed information (this type of information can be included in a secondary page).

TABLE 12.4—RECOMMENDATIONS ON WEB DESIGN AND USABILITY

General Guidelines for Web Site Design
  Set and state goals
  Tailor site to target audience(s)
  Create and evaluate prototypes
  Provide resources for Web site maintenance

Specific Layout and Navigation Techniques
  Use inverse pyramid approach for each page and section
  Include secondary pages for more extensive background information
  Write scannable and succinct text
  Keep navigation aids consistent and text-based (when possible)
  Limit page size
  Use readable fonts
  Use familiar fonts
  Indicate internal vs. external links
  Show used links
  Avoid using graphic links

Other Considerations
  Place sponsor name on each page
  Include a short index for commonly searched topics
  Provide a search engine if the site has >100 pages
  Provide text formatted printing options

Adapted from Reference 35

Text should be as succinct as possible and easily scannable, as most users scan Web site text rather than reading material in detail. It is essential to remember that writing for the Web is different than writing for other media. A general rule is to include no more than half of the text that would have appeared in a hard copy version. This may require dividing long blocks of text in short sentences or paragraphs that focus on a specific topic; such a structure allows users to easily find topics they are interested in and to download those segments. To get and maintain readers' attention, and to handle the tendency of readers to scan materials, Web pages should include simple but meaningful headlines, highlighted (bolded) and colored text, and visual images.

Links with titles in hypertext should be provided to allow users to readily access related Web sites. Graphics (visual images) often provide important breaks in text but must load quickly. Web sites must be readily and consistently navigable; users should be capable of easily viewing the material on each page, moving from page to page, locating information through indexes or hyperlinks, and linking to related Web sites. Well-designed sites load quickly so that users do not have to wait long.

If target audiences include persons with physical disabilities (impaired hearing or vision, for instance) or those who have access only through older technology,[33] then designers need to take these into account by modifying their sites. This may include approaches such as text-only versions of materials or inclusion of multi-media presentations. Text equivalents can also be used to describe the function or purpose of content for nontextual information (images or sounds). Text is considered accessible to almost all users because screen readers, nonvisual browsers, and Braille readers can handle it. There are federal regulations (i.e., Section 508) to make information technology more accessible; practitioners should consult laws or regulations applicable to their individual work situations.[34]

Other considerations for designing effective Web sites include using a short index for commonly searched topics, providing a search engine if a site has more than 100 pages, carefully pre-testing the design layout with the intended audience (formative evaluation), and providing resources to maintain sites.

Web design is rapidly becoming a specialized field within both informatics and communication, and consultation with experts is advised if practitioners will be designing or revising sites. Additional information on Web design and usability are available from the National Cancer Institute (usability.gov; reference 35) as well as in references 12 and 13.

LIMITATIONS OF ELECTRONIC COMMUNICATION

In addition to its benefits, electronic communication has a number of challenges as well. These include accessibility problems for certain populations such as persons with lower socioeconomic status or residents in rural areas (the "digital divide"),[5,36] reaching persons with low literacy or who are unfamiliar with computers,[37-42] rapidly changing hardware and software requirements resulting in disparities in technical capacity, privacy and confidentiality of information,[43,44] overuse of e-mail, locating appropriate Web sites, quality of Web site information,[2,21] assurance of information security,[45] and maintenance.

Electronic communication can reduce or eliminate printing costs and make materials more rapidly available by posting them on Web sites or by distributing them on CD-ROMs, but there may unintended consequences. Audiences may be less inclined to obtain or read materials distributed electronically that were previously available in print. Making materials available only in electronic forms may not achieve desired communication goals for many audiences, even those without access problems.

SUMMARY

Electronic communication is a powerful channel for rapidly transmitting written, audio, and visual information to audiences. E-mail and Web sites are the most common forms of electronic communication in public health practice. Electronic communication can rapidly reach large numbers of persons and facilitate new networks of people, yet it can be used to individualize communication efforts. Some of the challenges include ensuring access and quality, addressing the needs of diverse audiences, and ensuring privacy and confidentiality.

The general uses for electronic communication for public health include information collection, information provision, network creation, and interventions. Because of its widespread use and misuse, it is important to carefully consider whether e-mail is the best channel for reaching the intended audience and to follow certain guidelines when sending messages. The quality of health-related Web sites is a major concern. Assessing quality requires evaluating the sponsor of the Web site, information content, site design, and other factors. It is likely that the impact and importance of electronic communication for public health will increase as people become more adept at using these media. On the other hand, e-mail overload may diminish the utility of e-mail for interpersonal communication. The history of fax machines is illustrative: receiving a fax was a notable event a decade ago and demanded immediate attention; today, fax machines often lay unattended.

The expected convergence of voice, mass media, and computer technologies will open up new health communication opportunities.[1] Interventions based on electronic communication are likely to proliferate, as will the need to evaluate and communicate findings to multiple audiences. Assessing and ensuring the quality of information on Web sites, given the vast array of sites already available, will take on increased importance. There will be increased demand for independent organizations or trusted health intermediaries, such as public health professionals, to provide guidance to the public and patients about quality sources of online health information.

CHAPTER 12 ENDNOTES

1. Eng TR. The eHealth Landscape: A Terrain Map of Emerging Information and Communication Technologies in Health and Health Care. Princeton, NJ: Robert Wood Johnson Foundation; 2001. Available at: http://www.rwjf.org. Date of access: June 22, 2002
2. Eng TR, Gustafson D, Henderson J, Jimison H, Patrick K, for the Science Panel on Interactive Communication and Health. Introduction to evaluation of interactive health communication applications. *Am J Prev Med.* 1999;16:10-15.
3. Chamberlain MA. New technologies in health communication: progress or panacea? *Am Behavior Scientist.* 1994;38:271-284.
4. *Websters II New Riverside Dictionary.* Rev ed. Boston, MA: Houghton Mifflin; 1996.
5. U.S. Department of Commerce. *A Nation On-line: How Americans Are Expanding Their Use of the Internet.* Washington, DC: U.S. Department of Commerce, Economics and Statistics Administration, National Telecommunications and Information Administration; 2002.
6. Dutton WH, Rogers EM, Jun S. Diffusion and social impact of personal computers. *Communication Res.* 1987;14:219-249.
7. Rogers EM. *Communication Technology: The New Media in Society.* New York: Free Press; 1986.
8. Public Health Functions Steering Committee. *Public Health in America.* Washington, DC: US Department of Health and Human Services; 1994.

9. Meriwether RA. Blueprint for a national public health surveillance system for the 21st century. *J Public Health Management Practice*. 1996;2:16-23.

10. O'Carroll PW. Beyond Odwalla: epidemic investigation in an on-line world. *Washington Public Health*. 1997;15:40-43.

11. Centers for Disease Control and Prevention. HIV-related knowledge and stigma—United States, 2000. *MMWR*. 2000;49:1062-1064.

12. Nielsen J. Designing *Web Usability: The Practice of Simplicity*. Indianapolis: New Riders; 2000.

13. Badre AN. *Shaping Web Usability: Interaction Design in Context*. Reading, MA: Addison-Welsey; 2001.

14. Rossi PH, Freeman HE, Lipsey MW. *Evaluation: A Systematic Approach*. 6th ed. Thousand Oaks, CA: Sage; 1999.

15. McGinnis JM, Deering MJ, Patrick K. Public health information and the new media: a view from the Public Health Service. In: Harris LM, ed. *Health and the New Media: Technologies Transforming Personal and Public Health*. Mahwah, NJ: Lawrence Erlbaum Associates; 1995:127-141.

16. Humphreys BL, Ruffin AB, Cahn MA, Rambo N. Powerful connections for public health: the National Library of Medicine and the National Network of Libraries of Medicine. *Am J Public Health*. 1999;89:1633-1636.

17. National Cancer Institute. Cancer Information. Available at: http://cancer.gov. Date of access: June 22, 2002.

18. Centers for Disease Control and Prevention web site: http://www.cdc.gov. Date of access: June 22, 2002.

19. Robinson TN. Community health behavior change through computer network health promotion: preliminary findings from Stanford Health-Net. *Comput Methods Programs Biomed*. 1989;30:137-144.

20. Strecher VJ, Kreuter M, Den Boer DJ, Kobrin S, Hospers HJ, Skinner CS. The effects of computer-tailored smoking cessation messages in family practice settings. *J Fam Pract*. 1994;39:262-270.

21. Science Panel on Interactive Communication and Health. *Wired for Health and Well-Being: the Emergence of Interactive Health Communication*. Eng TR, Gustafson DH, eds. Washington DC: US Department of Health and Human Services; 1999.

22. Agency for Health Care Policy and Research(AHCPR). *Consumer Health Informatics and Patient Decision-Making. Final Report*. Rockville, MD: US Department of Health and Human Services, Agency for Health Care and Policy Research; 1997: AHCPR publication no. 98-N001.

23. Gottesman BZ. Take control of your e-mail. *PC Magazine*. May 5, 1998:101-107.

24. Search Engine Watch. Available at: http://www.searchenginewatch.com. Date of access: June 22, 2002.

25. The Spider's Apprentice. Available at: http://www.monash.com. Date of access: June 22, 2002.

26. Virtual Sites. Available at: http://www.virtualfreesites.com. Date of Access: June 22, 2002.

27. Medical World Search. Available at: http://www.mwsearch.com. Date of access: June 22, 2002.

28. Google search appliance: http://www.google.com. Date of access: February 23, 2002.

29. Lawrence S, Giles CL. Searching the World Wide Web. *Science*. 1998;280:98-100.

30. Kim P, Eng TR, Deering MJ, Maxfield A. Published criteria for evaluating health-related Web sites: review. *BMJ*. 1999; 318:647-649.

31. Winker MA, Flanagin A, Chi-Lum B, White J, Andrews K, Kennett RL et al. Guidelines for medical and health information sites on the Internet: Principles governing AMA Web sites. *JAMA*. 2000;283:1600-1606.

32. Federal Trade Commission. "Operation Cure.all" Targets Internet Health Fraud. Washington DC: Press release, June 24, 1999.

33. World Wide Web Consortium. Web Content Accessibility *Guidelines 1.0*. Boston, MA: World Wide Web Consortium. 1999. Available at: http://www.w3.org. Date of access: June 22, 2002.

34. Federal Rehabilitation Act (Section 508) requirements. Available at: http://www.section508.gov. Date of access: June 22, 2002

35. National Cancer Institute. *Evidence-Based Guidelines on Web Design and Usability*. Available at: http://usability.gov/guidelines/index.html. Date of access; June 22, 2002.

36. US Department of Commerce. *Falling Through the Net II: New Data on the Digital Divide*. Washington, DC: National Telecommunications and Information Administration; 1998. *37*.

37. Williams MV, Parker RM, Baker DW, Parikh NS, Pitkin K, Coates WC, et al. Inadequate functional health literacy among patients at two public hospitals. *JAMA*. 1995;274:1677-1682.

38. Baker DW, Parker RM, Williams MV, Pitkin K, Parikh NS, Coates W, et al. The health care experience of patients with low literacy. *Arch Fam Med.* 1996;5:329-334.
39. Yom SS. The Internet and the future of minority health. *JAMA.* 1996;275:735.
40. Williams MV, Baker DW, Parker RM, Nurss JR. Relationship of functional health literacy to patients' knowledge of their chronic disease: A study of patients with hypertension and diabetes. *Arch Intern Med.* 1998;158:166-172.
41. World Wide Web Consortium. *Web Accessibility Initiative (WAI).* Boston, MA: World Wide Web Consortium. Available at: http://www.w3.org. Date of access: June 22, 2002.
42. Graber MA, Roller CM, Kaeble B. Readability levels of patient education material on the World Wide Web. *J Fam Pract..* 1999;48:58-61.
43. National Research Council Computer Science and Telecommunication Board. *For the Record: Protecting Electronic Health Information.* Washington, DC: National Academy Press; 1997.
44. California HealthCare Foundation. *Americans Worry About the Privacy of Their Computerized Medical Records.* Oakland, CA: California HealthCare Foundation, January 28, 1999.
45. Stone B. Bitten by love. *Newsweek.* May 15, 2000; pp. 42.

SUGGESTED READINGS AND RESOURCES

Agency for Health Care Policy and Research (AHCPR). *Consumer Health Informatics and Patient Decision-Making. Final Report.* Rockville, MD: US Department of Health and Human Services, Agency for Health Care and Policy Research; 1997: AHCPR Pub. No. 98-N001.

Eng TR. The eHealth Landscape: A Terrain Map of Emerging Information and Communication Technologies in Health and Health Care. Princeton, NJ: Robert Wood Johnson Foundation; 2001. Available at: http://www.rwjf.org. Date of access: June 22, 2002.

Science Panel on Interactive Communication and Health. *Wired for Health and Well-Being: the Emergence of Interactive Health Communication.* Eng TR, Gustafson DH, eds. Washington DC: US Department of Health and Human Services; 1999.

Winker MA, Flanagin A, Chi-Lum B, White J, Andrews K, Kennett RL et al. Guidelines for medical and health information sites on the Internet: Principles governing AMA Web sites. *JAMA.* 2000;283:1600-1606.

Chapter Thirteen

RISK COMMUNICATION

Tim Tinker, DrPH, MPH
Elaine Vaughan, PhD

For public health practitioners, explaining and describing risk is probably the most challenging situation for communicating with nonscientists. The critical role of risk communication was never more evident than during the anthrax attacks in the fall of 2001. Unexpected and involuntary exposures to potential health hazards such as chemical or infectious agents, or concerns about the safety of pharmaceutical products or vaccines, are not uncommon in public health. Conflicting risks and messages, difficulty translating scientific information, media attention, and disagreement on the extent of the risk and how to assess it present difficult challenges.[1] Widespread fear and conflict among involved parties are common in such situations. This chapter is designed to help public health practitioners understand the principles and application of risk communication.

BACKGROUND

In a growing number of public and private sector agencies and organizations, risk communication is no longer an unfamiliar, technical term. Although the concept itself is still new to some, the abundance of conferences, seminars, and research studies on risk communication reflects the growing attention devoted to this topic. Risk communication activities are primarily the responsibility of employees in government agencies.

West Nile virus, Love Canal, anthrax, radiation from nuclear weapons tests, Legionnaire's disease, pesticide residues on fruit, silicone breast implants, flammable infant clothing, prescription diet pills, L-tryptophan, and mercury in childhood vaccines are just a few of many examples demonstrating the need for effective risk communication.

At the federal and state level, health, environmental, occupational, food and drug safety, energy, and consumer product safety agencies have been on the front line of risk communication for many years. For public and private agencies and organizations, risk communication efforts are generally motivated by a requirement for or desire to inform and involve the public; increase public trust and credibility; address public opposition to decisions; share power between government and public groups; and develop effective alternatives to direct regulatory control.

The many terms used in the subject area of risk can be confusing. Risk assessment is the process of organizing and evaluating information about the nature, strength of evidence, and likelihood of adverse health or ecological effects from particular exposures.[2] Risk management is the process of analyzing, selecting, implementing, and evaluating actions to reduce risk.[2] Stakeholders are the involved parties, such as individuals or organizations that are concerned about, or are affected by, the risk management problem.[2] Finally, risk communication is the interactive process of exchange of information and opinion among individuals, groups, and institutions. It involves providing messages about the nature of risk, as well as other messages that express concerns, opinions, or reactions to risk messages or to legal and institutional arrangements for risk management.[2]

Effective risk communication involves more than merely explaining a health or environmental risk to the public. A study on the communications policies and practices of federal agencies identified four general types of risk communications tasks: (1) information and education, (2) behavior change and protective action, (3) disaster warning and emergency information, and (4) joint problem solving and conflict resolution.[3]

What is needed at the core of risk communication is a solid understanding of stakeholders' needs, expectations, and priorities. There needs to be a multi-component strategy to address the public's concerns, to establish trust, and to alleviate fear and anger directed toward the person or organization considered responsible as well as towards government agencies. Finally, the public needs to be encouraged to participate in public health-related activities and in the decision-making process.[3,4]

Risk communication policies and practices among government agencies and private organizations tend to follow a more traditional public health orientation. The Environmental Protection Agency (EPA), for example, has taken the lead among federal environmental agencies in building risk communication into its regulatory policy activities and research agenda. A somewhat different version of risk communication has been embraced by the public health community, as many public health officials view risk communication as a tool for educating the public about health risks.[5]

These varying perceptions and approaches to health risk communication can be attributed in part to the diversity in mission, mandate, program focus, and culture. Approaches to risk communication often depend on whether the primary agency role is to regulate, conduct research, advise, or to resolve specific risk problems. Environmental protection agencies, which tend to have closer ties to the engineering community, approach problem-solving very differently from health agencies, which typically use a medically-oriented approach.[6-9] As a result of these different approaches, environmental agencies tend to have a "fix-it" mentality, while the "helping" tradition dominates in health agencies.[8]

In general, risk communication programs can be grouped into one of three broad categories: (1) disease prevention related to health risk behaviors,[10,11] (2) occupational and environmental exposures to toxic chemicals, and (3) product safety and consumer protection.[12] Risk communication is most often associated with exposure resulting in the onset of cancer or other chronic diseases, but it also applies to potentially acute or catastrophic situations such as the possibility of explosion or injury. Risk communication is also used in other public health arenas such as vaccine safety or potential risk of infectious diseases (for example, needle stick injuries to health care workers, bioterrorism, encephalitis).

Risk communication related to individual health risk behaviors has been extensively covered elsewhere and is beyond the scope of this book (see, for example, reference 11). The remainder of this chapter discusses risk communication and uses examples primarily drawn from environmental or occupational health settings, but most of these recommendations are applicable to other risk communication situations.

RISK PERCEPTION

Considerable research and experience points to a lack of understanding between the sender of a health risk message, such as a government agency, and the receiver of the message, such as the public.[13] Typically, a public health agency, when confronted with a potential health hazard, responds by examining the public health implications of the science and then works within its legal and economic constraints to provide its best assessment of the situation. That analysis, often presented in technical and uncertain terms, is sometimes poorly received by a public that demands certainty, is resistant to change, and is particularly sensitive to involuntary risks which they perceive as imposed on them by others (e.g., exposures to hazardous substances).

Unfortunately, when employees of a government agency do not understand and deal effectively with public perception of health risk, there is usually an increase in public concern about the risk and increased hostility toward the government agency.[4] Agency credibility suffers and the public becomes skeptical or indifferent to the information about health risks provided by agency experts. Poor health risk communication may also lead to ineffective public health interventions. Because agency assessments of health risk and public concerns do not correlate, some public health concerns go relatively unaddressed while others often command a disproportionate amount of agency resources.

"Hazardous activity" in the public's mind may include a wide range of events or activities that they determine to be "risky." To the scientist, however, hazard has a technical meaning and may not be associated with risk. To clarify the distinction, think of the technical portion of risk as hazard, and the nontechnical portion as "outrage;" scientists focus on "hazard," while concerned communities tend to focus more on outrage.[14,15] While the scientist sees risk determination as a technical process, the public sees it as a personal decision process. Table 13.1 compares views of scientists and the general public with respect to risk.[16]

If the public perceives that a risk exists, it is not uncommon for them to localize and personalize the situation. Community residents will often look to public health authorities for confirmation of their beliefs or decisions; they can become frustrated when a scientist's report does not confirm their beliefs or decisions or provides compelling evidence to the contrary. Practitioners should be aware that they cannot successfully communicate risk information to the general public in one or two meetings. Technical information on risk needs to be slowly digested by the general public audiences. Practitioners need to respond to questions to the best of their ability and follow up is essential.

Because the risk communication process is so deeply embedded in broader social issues, there are many barriers and problems.[4] A key barrier is the term "risk" itself–how is it measured, how is it described, and how is it perceived? Interested parties perceive risk different-

TABLE 13.1—DIFFERENCE IN THE APPROACH OF SCIENTISTS AND THE GENERAL PUBLIC TO RISK

Approach of Scientists	Approach of General Public
Trust in scientific methods and evidence	Trust in political culture and democratic process
Appeal of authority and expertise	Intuitive mental and perceptual models
Boundaries of analysis are narrow and reductionist	Boundaries of analysis are broad, and include the use of analogy and historical precedent
Risks are depersonalized	Risks are personalized
Emphasis on statistical variation and probability	Emphasis on the impacts of risk on family and community
Appeal to consistency and universality	Focus on particularity (individual situation) and less concerned about consistency of approach
When there is controversy in science, the status quo is maintained	When there is scientific controversy, public will decide which "side" to believe
Those impacts that cannot be measured are less relevant	Unanticipated or unarticulated risks are relevant

Adapted from References 5 and 16

ly, and people do not believe that all risks are of the same type, size, or importance. Table 13.2 provides examples of perceived "less risky" and "more risky" situations and related social equity issues.[17]

The perceptions of risk for the technical and lay audience are often dissimilar.[18] For example, a scientist may use a one-in-a-million comparison to convey a specific risk measurement. Other scientists understand this to mean that, given one million persons, there is one person who is at risk. To the non-technical person, however, the one person may be someone they know. The public will often personalize risk with the same conviction that most scientists depersonalize it.

Ultimately, the public will decide how much risk is acceptable, and their decision will be based on personal factors. One goal for the public health practitioner should be to educate

TABLE 13.2—THE GENERAL PUBLIC'S PERCEPTION OF RISK AND EQUITY

Less Risky	More Risky
Voluntary: Drive a car	*Involuntary:* Chemical plant in the neighborhood
Familiar: Household cleaners	*Unfamiliar:* A new incinerator
Natural: Radon in basement	*Man Made:* Chemicals made in a laboratory
Fair	**Unfair**
Controlled by self: Public invites	*Controlled by others:* Government forces new sewage plant new facility into the community onto a community
Not Memorable: Slow seepage of a chemical into the groundwater	*Memorable:* Fire

Adapted from Reference 17

the public on the level of risk and competing risks. Selling a community on acceptable risk may be difficult because people would prefer to live without environmental or technological risks whatsoever. However, by listening to and addressing concerns, the target audience will be better able to understand and, possibly accept, the risk.

PURPOSE, AUDIENCE, AND MESSAGE

As stressed throughout this book, practitioners must have a clear understanding of the purpose (why) of the communication, the audience (who), and the fundamental message (what) before doing risk communication.

Practitioners first must know the purpose, or why, of the risk communication. The initial impetus behind risk communication is usually reactive; that is, a health concern is raised, but depending upon the situation, risk communication activities can be either reactive or proactive. If communication about risk is to take place, is the goal to inform or persuade audiences? Each situation is unique, but with few exceptions, risk communication is used to assist individuals or policy makers with informed decision-making; for example, communicating the possible risk associated with exposure to product A.

Knowledge about the intended audience (who) is essential. It may be necessary to communicate risk to multiple audiences, including scientists, health care providers, patients, the general public, mass media representatives, administrators, private organizations, administrators, and elected officials. Messages need to be tailored for each of these audiences, and different channels may be necessary to reach different audiences (Box 13.1). Because of the complexity and uncertainty of the scientific issues, literacy and numeracy of audiences are especially important considerations if the target audience is to understand the message.[19,20] Communicating appropriately with the news media is especially critical in risk communication situations (chapter 6).

Creating messages constitutes the "what" of risk communication. Based on the science, purpose, audience, and situation, practitioners must decide on the main message to communicate. In risk communication this could be that there is "little reason for concern," "a great need for concern," or that "the potential risk is unknown." Planning is essential in

---

BOX 13.1

Exposure to radioactive materials can cause adverse health effects such as thyroid cancer. Several years ago it was discovered that residents living near Hanford, Washington, may have been exposed to the radioactive isotope Iodine-131. Federal agencies designed a multi-year scientific study to estimate the radiation exposure from Iodine-131 in the area.[21]

The Centers for Disease Control and Prevention (CDC) undertook a proactive communication effort to inform residents about the purpose, process, and results of the study. Before the report was released, CDC developed a public handbook to describe the study and to explain how radiation reaches people. After the report was released, the relevant government agencies had many public meetings and informal discussions with residents in the area to address public concerns and mistrust of government, and lay the groundwork for communicating study results. Risk communication efforts were designed to explain the project and the scientific uncertainties.

To build trust and credibility with the local community, several agencies developed a series of activities, including an ongoing local lecture series, small-group sessions, creation of fact sheets and educational materials, an 800 telephone number, media outreach, and open meetings of the technical steering committee. Surveys were also conducted to gauge the level of understanding and support for the project.

developing and using consistent messages, and a clear communication chain of command is necessary to avoid sending multiple and possibly conflicting messages.[3,4] Because of uncertainty and possibility of uncovering new information, recognize that the risk communication message may change over time.

MESSAGE PRODUCTION AND DELIVERY

Message production and delivery are major issues in risk communication. The choice of communication format, communication channels, and spokespersons depends on the specific situation, audience, and level of interest. Often, oral presentations or small group meetings with policy makers or individuals in affected communities are necessary to effectively address questions, fears, and anger that can occur in risk communication situations.

The timing (when) of the risk communication is important. Each situation will be different: sometimes there may be a need to communicate rapidly because of widespread concern (Box 13.2), while in other situations, delaying communication may be necessary for fear of creating unwarranted concern.

RECOMMENDATIONS FOR RISK COMMUNICATION

Good risk communication is often a complex endeavor with multiple perspectives, approaches, and components. The general principles that apply to most risk communication situations are outlined below.

REALIZE THAT EACH SITUATION IS UNIQUE

There is no ordinary risk communication situation.[3,4] The involved parties may live in geographic proximity or be scattered throughout the country. The type of exposure, extent, potential health risks, involved parties, and possible actions are highly variable and each situation is unique. As such, there are no pre-established rules or protocols, so the risk communication process needs to be flexible and unique to each situation; a "one size fits all" approach is a prescription for failure.

BOX 13.2

In 1990, the Food and Drug Administration (FDA) was informed by a manufacturer that the company planned to conduct a patient-notification program for an estimated 23,000 persons in the United States who received defective heart valves with potential deadly consequences.[22] The manufacturer planned to establish a program to locate affected patients, explain the problem, and recommend possible actions to be taken.

Attempts to identify and notify patients were undertaken through two methods: (1) media outreach, e.g., press conferences, news releases, and lay and professional journal advertisements; and (2) letters of notification to patients and physicians describing problems and risks. FDA staff participated in this risk communication effort by reviewing the manufacturer's patient notification letter. Initial versions of the letter lacked clarity and contained frightening messages, so the FDA facilitated the convening of focus groups of affected patients. Information obtained from these groups and from risk communication experts was used to create an improved notification letter.

A subsequent evaluation showed the letter to be a highly effective risk communication strategy: most recipients reported receiving and understanding the letter, and a majority felt relieved rather than irritated or frightened after reading it.

ASSESS SCIENTIFIC EVIDENCE

A critical element is the science behind risk communication activities and messages. Risk assessment is the scientific means to evaluate the extent of the health hazard to individuals and populations.[18,23] Although even with risk assessment there often remains much uncertainty, without it the recommendations, decisions, and actions will be based solely on opinion.

A comprehensive guide to conducting risk assessment is beyond the scope of this book; however, public health practitioners must carefully evaluate the quality of the information and the conclusions from risk assessment prior to developing their own conclusions and making recommendations. A staged or stepwise approach to risk assessment using a systematic protocol is commonly used by public health agencies to respond to possible outbreaks or clusters.[24] Such protocols usually specify when risk communication to affected individuals should occur. Persons conducting risk communication activities need to work closely with those involved in risk assessment to determine if or when risk communication should occur and message content. Ultimately, it is the risk communicator's responsibility to ensure that risk information and messages are based on the best available science and practice.

CONSIDER WHETHER RISK COMMUNICATION IS WARRANTED

Government agencies are often faced with the difficult problem of knowing when scientific information warrants risk communication. Integral to this question is the quality of the scientific information available to the agency. How reliable is the information; is it good enough to support a risk communication effort? Factors such as interpersonal contact, organizational culture and norms, intricate communication feedback loops, and the multiplicity of good and bad decisions will influence if and how health risk communication should occur.

RECOGNIZE AND ADDRESS AUDIENCE FEAR AND ANGER

Persons who find themselves potentially at risk for an adverse and involuntarily-imposed health problem are understandably fearful and angry. While uncertainty is a well-established part of science, most people are afraid of unknown risks and are inclined to focus on worst-case scenarios. As discussed previously, the concept of risk is far different if oneself, one's family members, or one's friends or neighbors are potentially affected compared to a random population elsewhere.[4] The involuntary nature of assuming any unknown health risk can easily exacerbate fears and generate much anger[15]. Failure to acknowledge and attempt to address the fear and anger of affected parties will likely result in unsuccessful risk communication and may increase concerns about an "government coverup."[3,4]

EXAMINE RISKS AND BENEFITS FROM MULTIPLE PERSPECTIVES

It is necessary to carefully consider who is at risk and who benefits in each risk situation. Fundamentally, most decisions about acceptable risk are not about risk at all but are a reflection of value judgments.[4] The environmental justice movement is an example of specific communities concerned about the differences between those who benefit and those who assume potential risk. Practitioners need a clear understanding of which populations experience the potential health risk and which stakeholders are responsible for the presence of the risk. In general, the party responsible for the existence of a potential risk derive some benefit. This benefit can result from the presence of the possible hazard itself or from not acting to eliminate the potential risk. The benefit is almost always financial (not paying for cleanup) for example, but in the case of a government agency being responsible (e.g., radiation from nuclear testing), it may be to avoid political embarrassment. It is also necessary to recognize that different government agencies may have vastly different perspectives on potential causes, willingness to share information, and actions to be taken.

If the potential hazard is eliminated, it is necessary to consider who would benefit from the action. Other specific considerations include the number of people who are at risk and the number who benefit, how long the benefits will last, and whether certain stakeholders receive a disproportionate share of the benefits.

INVOLVE STAKEHOLDERS IN THE PROCESS

Involving stakeholders, and especially the public, in the information-gathering process makes communications more credible and sets the stage for public participation in helping to resolve the problem.[16] Community residents, site personnel, citizen groups, health professionals, and state and local government representatives are all unique sources of information used by the risk communicator to relay public health and environmental risks. They can provide information concerning background information, community health concerns, demographics, and health outcomes.

Members of the general public need and want to be actively involved in identifying, characterizing, and solving problems that affect their lives.[4] Conducting open meetings, committing to an ongoing relationship with stakeholders, and providing names and phone numbers of experts that those affected community members can contact for help in better defining potential health implications can act to increase trust.

If a high level of credibility exists, stakeholders are more likely to believe the accuracy and completeness of the information provided. Uncertainty about information should be mentioned before the audience brings it up; audiences are more likely to accept uncertainty if a high level of trust has been achieved through a history of open and honest relationships.

A final note of caution is that public health practitioners should not involve stakeholders unless they are willing to be guided by their input: stakeholder involvement does not mean directing stakeholders to do what they are told to do.[25]

PROVIDE ADEQUATE RESOURCES AND USE PERSONS TRAINED IN RISK COMMUNICATION

To have success in risk communication, employees of government agencies and other involved parties must devote sufficient resources to stakeholder involvement and risk communication rather than simply consider such activities as an afterthought.[25] Unfortunately, there are many examples of poor risk communication. Providing resources refers not only to financial but to human resources as well by allowing employees to continue their involvement with stakeholders through attendance at meetings and responding to requests for further information. Furthermore, to make the process work the organization must have personnel trained and committed to making risk communication activities, especially in acute situations that receive extensive media attention.

ACKNOWLEDGE UNCERTAINTY

Recognizing and admitting uncertainty is simply the reality of most risk communication situations.[3,4] Unfortunately, revealing scientific uncertainty is a complicated point when trying to satisfy the demands of the public and mass media for reliable and meaningful information for many hazards and risks. Practitioners are frequently faced with the dilemma of having to acknowledge and explain uncertainty to a public who perceives scientific findings as precise, repeatable, and reliable. Moreover, the public often associates correlation as being the same as causality. As a result, practitioners are faced with the difficult task of trying to explain what their scientific data mean, as well as their limitations and uncertainties.

If information about risk is not known or not available, the best thing to do is to admit it. Although saying "I don't know" can evoke feelings of vulnerability, it can also be an important step in gaining credibility. If an audience demands 100% certainty, they are more than likely questioning the underlying values and process, not the science. By listening and recognizing the real concerns behind the demand for certainty, practitioners often can address audience fears while still acknowledging uncertainty. Audiences need to be provided as much information as possible to help them understand that uncertainty is part of the process and that the answers available now may not be the final answers.

TRANSLATE THE SCIENCE

When discussing risk, the focus should not be only on the health or environmental risk;[16] the importance of exposure paths may also need to be explained. For example, if the public hears over and over about a contaminant in their community and never fully understand how exposure occurs and who has been or may be exposed, convincing them later that they are not in danger may be impossible. Involve the public in discussions of exposure pathways. This will help them understand their risk and how to avoid or reduce their exposure to risk; it will also tap into their knowledge of potential exposure pathways that may not have been considered by the public health practitioner.

Scientific information will be more useful to the audience, and greater communication success will be achieved, if the information provided is relevant and easily understood.[16,26] To help audiences understand the issues, create well-targeted messages, use clear, non-technical language to discuss risks, exposure pathways, and other specific information concerning the nature, form, severity, or magnitude of the risk.

There are many ways to help with effective communication of complex scientific or technical information. Use consistent chemical names, groups of chemicals, units of measure, and other terms throughout a project—switching from parts per million to parts per billion can result in alarm because the higher numbers may be noticed but not the unit of measure. Avoid acronyms and jargon (such as ADI, SNARL, excess lifetime cancer risk) and provide careful definitions in advance. Carefully consider what information to include in tables and graphs, be sure all information is explained fully, and use these visuals to clarify and support key communications points.

Use familiar frames of reference to explain "how much" and create a mental picture of "parts per billion" or "tons per day" (numeric analogies). Reporting that the United States produces enough garbage in a day to fill 100 football fields 14 feet deep is much more meaningful than talking about 250,000 tons of garbage per day. However, examples should not be trite or condescending; take the time to develop meaningful examples and calculations. Answer not only the question "How much?" but also the question "Will it hurt me?" to ensure the information is relevant. For example, one way to do this would be to say that "At this site, we would expect that among 1 million people who drink about 8 ounces of water per day their entire lives, 1 person may get cancer caused by contaminants in the water, although this person may not necessarily die of cancer."[26]

Sometimes it may be helpful to indicate the level of certainty ("We are 95% certain, but we are conducting more studies to improve the accuracy"), but recognize that many non-scientific audiences such as the general public and the news media do not comprehend uncertainty in numeric terms and that this may require much explanation.

DESCRIBE SPECIFIC ACTIONS BEING TAKEN AND RECOMMEND ACTIONS FOR THE AUDIENCE

For nonscientific audiences, the primary concern is not the numbers but the actions being taken to reduce, prevent, or mitigate exposure to risk. Be specific about what is being done to find answers, and whenever possible, involve the community in efforts to solve the problem. It is equally important to provide an explanation as to how the research is being done and why it may take some time before the answers are available. A distinction should be made between areas of scientific uncertainty and uncertain responses because of lack of science.

In addition to the actions being taken by government agencies, businesses, and other parties, potentially exposed individuals need information on the actions that they can take. For example, what can they do to discover if they have been exposed, if they may be at increased risk, or actions that they should take to reduce risk? Examples of actions for exposed individuals could include providing names of people or phone numbers for further information, reducing or eliminating the use of a product, or consulting with a health care provider.

CHALLENGES AND BARRIERS

LACK OF SCIENTIFIC CONSENSUS

In the ideal world, risk assessment will provide clear-cut answers and the scientific community would reach consensus about the extent of risk and the actions to be taken. As mentioned throughout the chapter, however, it is common to have scientific uncertainty about whether there is increased risk or the potential benefits of specific actions designed to reduce that risk (especially in environmental and occupational health). For chronic diseases such as cancer, health effects based on high levels of exposure in humans or animals are often extrapolated to estimate health effects at lower levels of exposure.[18]

Even more difficult are situations in which well-respected scientific experts disagree about risks, benefits, or proposed solutions.[27] Science and scientists are not value-free,[28] and each scientist has his or her beliefs about what constitutes an acceptable risk, benefit, or solution. This lack of consensus makes formulating risk communication messages especially difficult.

RISK COMPARISONS

Risk comparisons are generally not helpful in risk communication and should usually be avoided.[3,15,29,30] Irrelevant or misleading comparisons can harm trust and credibility, and inappropriate comparisons can make situations worse. Comparing the chance of becoming ill from a chemical exposure to the chance of being hit by lightning, for example, would be counterproductive in a community in which someone actually had been hit by lightning. Comparisons may also be confusing or even insulting to individuals who weigh risks not only on the probability that a disastrous event will occur, but also on whether they choose to take the risk and how much control they believe they have over the situation.

If practitioners decide to use risk comparisons, several recommendations are listed in Table 13.3. Factors other than the relative risk of one exposure compared to another need to be acknowledged as important. If comparisons are used, the safest comparison is to a government standard (but the meaning of the standard must be explained), and the comparisons used to clarify, rather than minimize, the risk. Comparisons should not be used in emotion-laden situations or to justify the benefits, nor should they be made between involuntary and voluntary risks (environmental chemical exposure compared with active cigarette smoking).

MAINTAIN NEUTRALITY

Affected or concerned individuals, corporation representatives, unions, advocacy groups, and government agencies often have widely divergent goals. Maintaining neutrality in risk communication situations is a difficult but essential task for practitioners. Because of the weight of the evidence, values, beliefs, conflicts of interest, or past experiences, public health practitioners may directly or indirectly favor one stakeholder over others. For example, a practitioner may have once been a union member, and as such, he/she may consider their role to be a worker advocate and seek to maximize the perceived potential risk when communicating with exposed individuals. In contrast, other practitioners may have a fatalistic outlook on life ("everything causes cancer")[4] and minimize the concerns of others about potential risks.

In the often highly charged environment of risk communication, neutrality must be maintained if public health practitioners are to develop ongoing and trusting relationships, have credibility, and move audiences to respond to communication messages. Minimizing a risk to reassure an alarmed community, or using alarming risks to arouse concern in an apathetic community, can both weaken credibility and appear more like manipulation than honest communication.[30]

MANAGE COMMUNICATION WITH THE NEWS MEDIA

Factors such as newness, geographic proximity, consequence, human interest, conflict, unusualness, injustice, blame, or controversy all act to increase the likelihood of news media interest.[31] Several, and sometimes all, of these factors are often present in risk communica-

---

TABLE 13.3—CONSIDERATIONS WHEN MAKING RISK COMPARISONS

Compare to an acceptable standard (government standard is safest)
Acknowledge that relevant factors beyond relative risk exist
Make comparisons to help clarify the issue rather than minimize or dismiss it
Do not compare risk if atmosphere is heavily laden with fear, anger, or blame
Do not use comparison of benefits to justify risks
Do not compare voluntary with involuntary risks

tion situations; as a consequence, such situations are often deemed newsworthy.

Developing a strategy for communicating risk communication information to the news media is essential. Controversy, blame, unsuspecting victims, and the unspoken hint of a "government coverup" can potentially generate many news stories; news media representatives can usually locate concerned individuals, company spokespersons, and independent experts to speak about the situation. Honesty, acknowledging uncertainty, message consistency (realizing that the message may change over time), and using spokespersons familiar with the news media can often reduce the potential media problems. Additionally, honesty and ongoing relationships with the media can help lower concerns among the general public when the risk assessment suggests minimal risk; the media can play a key role as an intermediary for encouraging specific actions by general public. (Further discussion about communicating with media representatives is covered in chapter 6.)

RISK COMMUNICATION PLANNING

Planning is essential for successful risk communication.[32,33] The risk communication plan should employ specific risk communication techniques and approaches rather than generic program goals; it should be based on a working knowledge of the affected population; provide a framework for addressing audience concerns; and, most of all, it should be flexible and allow for the unexpected. Revisions and updates should be made as needed to keep the approach current and relevant.

Communication planning efforts should be designed to cover a wide range of community concerns about the cause, magnitude, and consequences of the specific risks; deliver messages through the appropriate individuals or intermediaries (e.g., community members, health care providers); and assess the quality and impact of risk communications activities based on community concerns and needs through careful evaluation.[32] Table 13.4 provides a list of background questions for assisting in communication planning in environmental situations, and Figure 13.1 contains a list of specific information to obtain and activities to conduct for risk communication efforts.

BIOTERRORISM AND COMMUNICATION

The information presented thus far in this chapter also applies to bioterrorist events, but the importance of good risk communication skills in such situations and the adverse effects of poor communication, are magnified considerably. [34] Bioterrorism can result in widespread fear, outrage, and elevated risk perceptions,[34] resulting in intense pressure on government officials to "do something." Poor communication can result in at-risk populations panicking, taking inappropriate actions, and losing trust in government officials or agencies.[35-38]

As evidenced by the anthrax attacks in 2001, a future bioterrorist event would inevitably involve multiple government agencies at the local, state, and federal levels, each with somewhat different roles and agendas, and would generate intensive and ongoing media scrutiny. Risk communication in such situations can be even more challenging for public health agencies when law enforcement agencies are involved. Law enforcement agencies are not inclined to share information or communicate with public health agencies or the mass media, especially if the information is uncertain, out of fear of jeopardizing criminal investigations.

Communication must be a central feature of responding to a bioterrorism event, and it can have multiple purposes.[34-36,39] These may include informing and instructing widely

TABLE 13.4—CONSIDERATIONS WHEN DEVELOPING RISK COMMUNICATION MESSAGES

Questions to Ask About the Extent of the Risk(s)
What are the hazards of concern?
What is the probability of exposure to each hazard?
What is the distribution of exposure?
What is the probability of each type of harm from a given exposure to each hazard?
What are the sensitivities of different populations to each hazard?
How do exposures interact with exposures to other hazards?
What are the qualities of the hazard?
What is the total population risk?

Questions to Ask About the Nature of the Benefits from the Exposure
What are the benefits associated with the hazard?
What is the probability that the projected benefit will actually follow the activity in question?
What are qualities of the benefits?
Who will benefit and in what way?
How many people benefit and how long do benefits last?
Which group get a disproportionate share of the benefits?
What is the total benefit?

Questions to Ask About Alternatives
What are the alternatives to the hazard in question?
What is the effectiveness of each alternative?
What are the risk and benefits of alternative actions and of not acting?
What are the cost and benefits of each alternative and how are they distributed?

Questions to Ask About Uncertainties in Risk Knowledge
What are the weaknesses of available data?
What are the assumptions on which estimates are based?
How sensitive are the estimates to change in assumptions?
How sensitive is the decision to change in the estimate?
What other risk and risk control assessments have been made and why are they different from those now being offered?

Questions to Ask On Managing Risk
Who is responsible for the decision?
What issues have legal importance?
What constrains the decision?
What resources are available?

Adapted from Reference 2

divergent audiences (the public, health care providers, news media); minimizing panic or fear; encouraging the adoption of appropriate protective actions by individuals; building trust; and minimizing or dispelling misinformation or rumors.[35,39,40]

FIGURE 13.1—QUICK PLANNING GUIDE TO
ENVIRONMENTAL RISK COMMUNICATION

Staff Plan
Form your communications response team. Think about the expertise and strengths each member brings to the team. Identify who will have what communications responsibilities. Members from outside the immediate team, such as community residents, should also be invited to participate in the planning process.

Name and phone number   *Responsibilities*
_____   _____
_____   _____
_____   _____
_____   _____
_____   _____

<None>
Summarize the risk problem or situation:_____
_____

Summarize the health risk situation:_____
_____

Audience's Concerns
What are the community's main concerns?
Health:_____
_____

Environmental:_____
_____

Economic:_____

Legal:_____
_____

Resources and Contacts
List the name, address, phone and e-mail for key contacts.
State Health Department: _____
_____

Local Health Department: _____

EPA Regional Department: _____

Other:_____
_____

Media
List the station/paper contact name, address, phone for the major media serving the community.
Newspaper: _____

Radio: _____

Television:_____
_____

Audiences
List the three main audiences, identify the key contact/s, and summarize the group's concerns.
1._____
_____
2._____
_____
3._____
_____

Objectives
Determine your risk communication objectives. Consider which behaviors, beliefs, and attitudes of the audience you want to influence.
1._____
2._____
3._____

Messages
Write out the three main messages. Once these are chosen, use them consistently.
1._____
2._____
3._____

Strategies and Techniques
Outline risk communication strategies (What is planned?) and tactics (How will it be achieved?).
1._____
Tactic:_____
Tactic:_____
2._____
Tactic:_____
Tactic:_____
3._____
Tactic:_____
Tactic:_____
4._____
Tactic:_____
Tactic:_____
5._____
Tactic:_____
Tactic:_____

Time Line
Create a time line for health risk communication activities, including the responsible party and due dates.

Evaluation
The plan should be outlined, including objectives, so that work done can be tracked.

Pretesting messages and materials with intended audience (formative evaluation) to help create best messages and delivery methods:

_____
_____

Process evaluation to review and document activities conducted:

_____
_____

Mid-point (outcome) evaluation to determine whether short-term objectives were met:

Results (impact) evaluation to assess long-term impact:

Understanding the psychological processes that people experience in such circumstances[37] can assist public health practitioners in their selection of appropriate communication strategies and message development for specific audiences. Intra-agency cooperation, coordination, and communication are essential to avoid the problem of agencies issuing multiple and potentially conflicting messages. It is essential to develop an effective strategy for communicating with the news media (chapter 6),[36,39] which must include carefully considering the selection of the spokesperson.

Advance planning and rehearsal by government agencies on how to handle communication in a bioterroism situation is critical.[36,39] Consultation with experts in risk communication experienced in crisis situations is strongly advised in the event of such an attack. (More detailed information on communication and bioterrorism can be found in references 34, 35, 36, 39, and 41, and at CDC's bioterrorism Web site, www.bt.cdc.gov).

SUMMARY

Risk communication is the interactive process of exchange of information and opinion among individuals, groups, and institutions. It requires understanding stakeholders' needs, expectations, and priorities, and developing strategies that address their concerns, establish trust, alleviate fear and anger, and encourage stakeholder participation in activities and decisions. There are substantial differences in risk perception between scientists and the general public that must be recognized and addressed. As in other communication situations, practitioners need to understand the purpose, audience, and message.

There are several recommendations for improving risk communication. These include realizing that each situation is unique; assessing the scientific evidence; considering whether communication is warranted; addressing audience fear and anger; examining risks and benefits from multiple perspectives; involving stakeholders in the process; acknowledging uncertainty; translating the science; and describing specific actions underway and the recommended course of actions for potentially affected individuals. Challenges include lack of scientific consensus, risk comparisons, need for neutrality, and managing communication to the news media. Careful planning and evaluation can greatly facilitate effective risk communication. Communication plays a central role in bioterrorism, and intra-agency cooperation, coordination, and communication are essential to avoid sending multiple and conflicting messages.

The need for public health practitioners to develop effective risk communication skills is likely to increase. Information previously available only to the scientific community will increasingly be available to nonscientists and communicated to other nonscientists through the Internet.[42] Involuntary chemical exposures,[34-36,39] infectious diseases, and consumer product safety concerns are often newsworthy, and given the growing number of media outlets available to the general public, reporters will continue to search for health risk-related stories. The increased use of certain forms of alternative and complementary medicine, reductions in the length of time it takes for pharmaceutical products to reach the market, increased opposition to immunizations, and concerns about bioterrorism are likely to increase the need and demand for effective risk communication.

CHAPTER 13 ENDNOTES

1. U.S. Department of Health and Human Services. Risk Communication: Working with Individuals and Communities to Weigh the Odds. *Prevention Report.* Washington, D.C,: February/March 1995:1-2.
2. National Research Council Commission/National Academy of Sciences. *Improving Risk Communication.* Washington, DC: National Academy Press; 1989.
3. Covello VT, McCallum DB, Pavlova M, eds. *Effective Risk Communication: The Role and Responsibility of Government and Nongovernment Organizations.* New York: Plenum Press; 1987.
4. Bennett P, Calman K eds. *Risk Communication and Public Health.* New York: Oxford; 1999.
5. Plough A, Krimsky S. *Environmental Hazards: Communicating Risks as a Social Process.* Westport, CT: Auburn House; 1988.
6. Chess C. Encouraging effective risk communication in government: suggestions for agency management. In: Covello VT, McCallum DB, Pavlova MT eds. *Effective Risk Communication: The Role and Responsibility of Government and Nongovernment Organizations.* New York: Plenum Press; 1987.
7. Chess C, Hance BI. Opening doors: making risk communication agency reality. *Environment* 1989;31:11-15.
8. Chess C, Sandman PM, Greenberg MR. *Empowering Agencies to Communicate About Environmental Risk: Suggestions for Overcoming Organizational Barriers.* New Brunswick, NJ: Environmental Communication Research Program, Rutgers University, 1990.
9. Chess C, Tamuz M, Saville A, Greenberg M. *The Organizational Links Between Risk Communication and Risk Management: The Case of Sybron Chemicals Inc.* New Brunswick, NJ: Environmental Communication Research Program, Rutgers University; 1991.
10. Roper WL. Health communication takes on new dimensions at CDC. *Public Health Rep.*1993;108:179-183.
11. Backer TE, Rogers EM. *Organizational Aspects of Health Communication Campaigns: What Works?* Newbury Park, CA: Sage; 1993.
12. Allen FW. The government as lighthouse: a summary of federal risk communication programs. In: Covello VT, McCallum DB, Paviova MT eds. *Effective Risk Communication: The Role and Responsibility of Government and Nongovernment Organizations.* New York: Plenum Press; 1987.
13. Agency for Toxic Substances and Disease Registry. *National Health Risk Communication Training Program for State Health Agency Personnel.* Atlanta, GA: ATSDR;1991.
14. Plough A, Krimsky S. The emergence of risk communication studies: social and political context. *Science Technol Human Values.* 1987;12:3-4.
15. Sandman P. *Responding to Community Outrage: Strategies for Effective Risk Communication.* Fairfax, VA: American Industrial Hygiene Association, 1993.
16. Slovic P, Fischoff B, Lichtenstein S. Facts and fears: understanding perceived risk. In: Schwing R and Albers WA Jr., eds. *Societal Risk Assessment: How Safe is Safe Enough?* New York: Plenum; 1980.
17. Frewer LJ. Public risk perceptions and risk communication. In: Bennett P, Calman K, eds. *Risk Communication and Public Health.* New York: Oxford; 1999.
18. Samet JM, Burke TA. Epidemiology and risk assessment. In: Brownson RC, Petitti DB, eds.: *Applied Epidemiology: Theory to Practice.* New York: Oxford; 1998.
19. Woloshin S, Schwartz LM, Moncur M, Gabriel S, Tosteson AN. Assessing values for health: numeracy matters. *Med Decis Making.* 2001;21:382-390.
20. Presidential/Congressional Commission on Risk Assessment and Risk Management. *Framework for Environmental Health Risk Management: Final Report* (Vol 1). Washington DC: Presidential/Congressional Commission on Risk Assessment and Risk Management; 1997.
21. Shipler DB, Napier BA, Farris WT, Freshley MD. Hanford environmental dose reconstruction project: an overview. *Health Physics.* 1996;71:532-544.
22. Chesley SM. Worldwide call for patients with Bjork-Shiley Convexo-Concave heart valve. *J Am Coll Cardiol.* 1992;19:1368.

23. Lundgren RE. *Risk Communication: A Handbook for Communicating Environmental, Safety and Health Risks.* Columbus, OH: Battelle Press, 1994.

24. Brownson RC. Outbreak and cluster investigations. In: Brownson RC, Petitti DB, eds. *Applied Epidemiology: Theory to Practice.* New York: Oxford University Press; 1998.

25. Sandman PM. Ethical considerations and responsibilities when communicating health risk information: emerging communication responsibilities of epidemiologists. *J Clin Epidemiol.* 1991;44(suppl 1):41S-50S.

26. Bean MC. Speaking of risk. *Civil Engineering.* 1988;58:60.

27. Taubes G. Epidemiology faces its limits. *Science.* 1995;269:164-169.

28. Krieger N. The making of public health data: paradigms, politics, and policy. *J Public Health Policy.* 1992;13:412-427.

29. Sandman PM, Miller PM, Johnson BB, Weinstein ND. Agency communication, community outrage, and perception of risk: Three simulation experiments. *Risk Analysis.* 1993;13:585- 598.

30. Sandman PM. Explaining risk to non-experts. *Emergency Preparedness Digest.* October-December 1987:25-29.

31. Wallack L, Dorfman L, Jernigan D, Themba M. *Media Advocacy and Public Health. Power for Prevention.* Newbury Park, CA: Sage Publications; 1993.

32. Tinker TL, Collins CM, King HS, Hoover MD. Assessing risk communication effectiveness: perspectives of agency practitioners. *J Hazardous Materials.* 2000; B73:17-27.

33. Pfugh KK, Shaw JA, Johnson BB. *Establishing Dialogue: Planning for Success.* Report to the New Jersey Department of Environmental Protection, Division of Science and Research. Trenton, NJ: New Jersey Department of Environmental Protection; 1992.

34. Ursano RJ, Fullerton CS, Fullerton AE, eds. *Planning for Bioterrorism.* New York: Cambridge University Press. In press.

35. Centers for Disease Control and Prevention. Biological and chemical terrorism: Strategic plan for preparedness and response: Recommendations of the CDC strategic planning workgroup. *MMWR.* 2000;49(RR-02):1-14.

36. Association of State and Territorial Directors of Health Promotion and Public Health Education. *Model emergency response communications plan for infectious disease outbreak and bioterrorist events.* Washington, DC: ASTDHPPHE Press; 2000.

37. National Research Council. *Understanding Risk: Informing Decisions in a Democratic Society.* Washington, DC: National Academy Press, 1996.

38. Slovic P. Trust, emotion, sex, politics and science: Surveying the risk-assessment battlefield. *Risk Analysis.* 1999;19:689-701.

39. Covello V, Peters RG, Wojtecki JG, Hyde RC. Risk communication, the West Nile Virus epidemic, and bioterrorism: responding to the communication challenges posed by the intentional or unintentional release of a pathogen in an urban setting. *J Urban Health: Bull NY Acad Med.* 2001;78:382-391.

40. DiGiovanni C. Domestic terrorism with chemical or biological agents: Psychiatric aspects. *Am J Psychiatry.* 2000;156:1500-05.

41. Sandman PM. Anthrax, bioterrorism, and risk communication: guidelines for action. Available at: http://psandman.com/ Date of Access: June 22, 2002.

42. Eng TR, Gustafson DH, eds. Science Panel on Interactive Communication and Health: *Wired for Health and Well-Being: the Emergence of Interactive Health Communication.* Washington DC: US Department of Health and Human Services; 1999.

SUGGESTED READINGS AND RESOURCES

Bennett P, Calman K, eds. *Risk Communication and Public Health.* New York: Oxford; 1999.

Cancer Risk Communication: What We Know and What We Need To Learn. *JNCI Monogr.* 1999;25:1-185.

Covello V, Peters RG, Wojtecki JG, Hyde RC. Risk communication, the West Nile Virus epidemic, and bioterrorism: responding to the communication challenges posed by the intentional or unintentional release of a pathogen in an urban setting. *J Urban Health: Bull NY Acad Med.* 2001;78:382-391.

Sandman PM. *Responding to Community Outrage: Strategies for Effective Risk Communication.* Fairfax, VA: American Industrial Hygiene Association; 1993.

Ursano RJ, Fullerton CS, Fullerton AE, eds. *Planning for Bioterrorism.* New York: Cambridge University Press; in press.

PART IV:

NEXT STEPS

Chapter Fourteen

FUTURE DIRECTIONS

David E. Nelson, MD, MPH
Jennifer A. Woodward, PhD
Ross C. Brownson, PhD
Patrick L. Remington, MD, MPH
Claudia Parvanta, PhD

R ecent changes in communication technology and the increasing volume of information provide an excellent opportunity to reexamine the roles of public health practitioners.[1-3] The assessment and policy development functions of public health require that information be effectively translated and communicated to inform or persuade policy makers and the general public to make individual- or policy-level changes.[4,5] Public health communication is especially germane for epidemiology, since the need to synthesize, translate, and communicate scientific information to different audiences has never been greater. Previous chapters have focused on helping public health practitioners improve their skills in these areas, and this chapter suggests future directions for improvement.

Effectively communicating public health information beyond the scientific community remains a challenge despite the recommendations discussed in this book. It requires practitioners to step out of the usual professional-to-professional communication model that is generally comfortable and safe. To improve the likelihood that more communication will occur between public health professionals and nonscientists, and that such communication activities will be of high quality, will require changes in at least six areas: health communication education and training; health communication research; coordination and utilization of existing public health knowledge; enhanced tailoring of messages and use of multiple media channels; improved cultural communication competency; and creating the infrastructure for equitable access and use of new communication technologies.

INCREASED HEALTH COMMUNICATION EDUCATION AND TRAINING

There is an ever growing need for public health students to be well-versed in the methods of health communication.[6,7] Although there are exceptions,[8] few schools offer extensive curricula in this field. Of all the public health disciplines, health education and health promotion have the strongest history of emphasizing communicating with nonscientific audiences, but courses often focus solely on reaching the public to promote individual health behavior change.[9,10]

Education needs to be broad-based and should include instructors from outside of the health arena, (journalism, communication, business, and political science). Recently, there has been increased awareness by the Association of the Schools of Public Health of the need for greater education of public health students in health communication.[11] Increased integration of the curricula of public health and communication is long overdue.

Training of the existing public health workforce in health communication is also needed.[3,7,12-20] As mentioned in chapter 1, the Council on Linkages Between Academia and Public Health Practice has issued a Consensus Set of Core Competencies that highlights the need for improved communication training for practitioners.[11] Findings from focus group interviews with state chronic disease program leaders highlighted the growing need for communication skills in the areas of management, epidemiology, and policy development.[3] University courses are an option for some practitioners, but a more viable alternative is short courses or institutes sponsored by universities, government agencies, or private organizations. With the development of distance-based learning via satellite broadcasts, interactive CD-ROMs, and the Internet, courses can be developed to reach broad audiences.

A few communication courses for public health practitioners are already in use. CDCynergy, developed by CDC, is a large step forward in attempting to use public health data and information to encourage public health action through improved communication.[21] CDCynergy is based on CD-ROM technology combined with a 3-day in-person training course. Attendees are taught to use a step-wise approach to review existing public health data and information, analyze audiences, develop messages, and select communication channels. It is an excellent tool for developing and planning; it does not, however, emphasize policy or advocacy approaches. The Tobacco Use Prevention Training Institute (TUPTI),[22] sponsored annually by CDC and the Robert Wood Johnson Foundation, trains public health professionals to communicate outside the scientific community on tobacco-related issues. In contrast to CDCynergy, this program is less formally structured and covers communication for policy and advocacy purposes.

Health communication education and training need not be limited to courses developed or sponsored by universities or the federal government. National, state, and local public health organizations, as well as state and local health departments, could assist in developing and sponsoring such training, through courses at the national and regional conferences. Coordination of education and training is needed to maximize the use of resources.

INCREASED HEALTH COMMUNICATION RESEARCH

There are many areas for which research is needed on communication in public health. The most obvious, but not necessarily the most important, is research on the impact and role that electronic communication can play in public health. For example, more than half of all Americans are Internet-users, and obtaining health information is one of the most common reasons for searching Web sites.[23-25] More research is needed on why individuals use the Internet to obtain health information, the quality of data and other information accessed, impact of information gathered from the Internet (changes in knowledge, behaviors, advocacy efforts, for example), ways to improve the presentation and availability of data and other information,[26] and counteracting misinformation are just a few of many examples.[27,28]

But there are more basic health communication research issues directly applicable to public health practice. There is a need to review and evaluate the utility of data for public health practice that are collected from the myriad of federal, state, and local surveillance systems, as well as the dissemination of information from these systems. Because of inertia, the conservative nature of governmental bureaucracies, and fear of criticism for not having obtained certain data items, few systems undergo a comprehensive review of the relevancy of the information obtained for advancing public health. Opportunity cost—the lost chance to obtain and disseminate different and potentially more valuable information—is seldom considered.

In 1988 Thacker outlined the key components of public health surveillance. The last element is "the dissemination and utilization of data to those who need to know."[29] In this seminal article, Thacker states that there has been little research on the dissemination and utilization of public health surveillance data. Unfortunately, little has changed; for example, among the sparse literature, two recent studies evaluated the utility and use of data collected in the Behavioral Risk Factor Surveillance System.[30,31] Literature reviews turned up few published evaluations on the utility of data obtained from surveillance systems.

There is limited research on the dissemination and use of public health information. For example, what are the best communication formats and channels for public health practitioners to communicate with certain audiences, such as the news media, elected officials, or private health organizations? There is a large "knowledge-generating" research establishment that often focuses on identifying new risk factors. In contrast, there is a very small "knowledge-use" research establishment, and much of its effort has concentrated on proactive campaigns, especially those directed toward mass media or individual change in limited research situations.

There is a great need for health communication research based on prospective experimental and quasi-experimental designs, time-series analyses, qualitative research, and even case studies that evaluate the dissemination and utilization of existing public health information. Such research is especially needed at the state and local-level. In addition, research is needed on how nonscientific audiences learn about public health information, the best formats for reaching different audiences, and how public health information is interpreted. Recently, the National Cancer Institute decided to make a major investment in health communication research by sponsoring the Centers of Excellence in Cancer Communications Research grant program.[32]

IMPROVED TRANSLATION OF EXISTING PUBLIC HEALTH INFORMATION

Coordinating, translating, and communicating existing health information is another large health communication issue. There are examples of how this is already being done for practitioners, such as the Surgeon General Reports on Tobacco[33] and Reports to Congress on Alcohol and Health.[34] Private and voluntary health organizations also routinely publish such information for topics under their purview.[35] The summary of information in the Guide to Clinical Preventive Services[36] and the Guide to Community Preventive Services[37] are also valuable for public health practitioners, as are reviews of some topics through the NIH Consensus Development Program[38] and reports by National Academy of Sciences.[39] One of the major challenges in coordinating, synthesizing, and translating health data is the large number of public health surveillance data sources. Most systems operate independently, especially those sponsored by different federal agencies, and this problem of multiple and independent data systems is commonly repeated at the state and local level because of categorical funding. Improved coordination of data collection, publication of information, and efficient dissemination of the information available from federal, state, and local agencies is essential. Fortunately, with the advent of Internet technology, linkage of Web sites across agencies is beginning to occur, as are Web site linkages between private health organizations and public health agencies.

Data and other information need to be published in formats readily available and understood by nonscientific audiences. The National Cancer Institute (NCI) and CDC have been leaders in providing information on their Web sites targeted specifically to certain populations such as practitioners, patients, and the news media.[40,41] Other federal agencies, as well as state and local agencies and voluntary health organizations, need to target their Web site materials to meet the needs of multiple audiences.

Much of the provision of public health information to the general public can only be considered as diffusion, that is, the "trickle-down" of information from researchers, individual agencies, and others. Research on understanding and improving the process of translating and disseminating public health information to various audiences is sorely needed. Woolf has suggested the creation of a national program, sponsored by government and private organizations, to synthesize evidence on health issues guiding policy development, as well as individual practices and programs.[42] To be most effective, this proposed national program must generate useful products and materials for scientific and nonscientific audiences alike.[42]

Given the explosion in information and information availability, more must be done to encourage and support persons trained to translate public health information, especially among those trained in epidemiology or the social sciences. For example, individuals capable of examining and evaluating public health-related Web sites are needed, as the quality of information at sites is highly variable.[23,28] Because of the explosion in the availability of data and other information, it may be time to consider developing a new public health specialty for translating public health information to nonscientific audiences.

ENHANCED TAILORING OF MESSAGES AND INCREASED USE OF MULTIPLE MASS MEDIA CHANNELS

The ongoing advancements in electronic communication and data systems technologies, along with the growing fragmentation of mass media, will provide challenges for public health practitioners attempting to reach the general public. Further refinements are on the horizon for enhanced tailoring of messages to more homogeneous and smaller audiences.[23] Until now, most tailoring has been based on relatively crude categories such as demographics and geographic location.[43] Given the crowded mass media environment and the increased choices people have in their selection of media,[23,44] practitioners will need to tailor public health messages by taking into consideration additional factors. Among these may be such things as preferred medium, culture, values, literacy, attentiveness to specific health topics, and timing (e.g., time of day, day of the week).[23]

Closely related to improved tailoring of messages will be the need to provide public health messages through multiple mass-media channels. Gone are the days when three major television networks provided national evening news to a large proportion of the population. Because of changes in television and the development of the Internet, people now have more media choices than ever before: access to hundreds of television stations (many with distinct audience niches) is available through cable or satellite systems, and interactive television already exists in some markets. The increased access to larger bandwidth (broadband) will likely lead to the development of even more user-centered systems.[23]

This fragmentation of mass media channels[44] affects the delivery of public health messages to the public. Practitioners can no longer assume that coverage of a public health story by a local newspaper or television station is sufficient to reach a large portion of the general population. To reach a substantial segment of the target audiences, health messages will have to be delivered several times through multiple media channels.

IMPROVED CULTURAL COMMUNICATION COMPETENCY

The diversity of the United States' population continues to change at a rapid pace. In the year 2000, an estimated 10% of Americans were born outside the U.S.[45] For many people, English is a second or even a third language.[46] Distinct subcultures based on immigrant populations from many continents exist throughout the country; Asian and Pacific Islanders, for example, consist of about 30 different linguistic and cultural groups.[47] Certain public health problems, such as tuberculosis, disproportionately affect specific immigrant populations,[48] making effective communication across cultures even more essential for practitioners.

Elevating the awareness of practitioners about cultural differences in communication, and increased training on how to create culturally appropriate messages, is crucial.[46] Many Asian cultures, for example, are based on a collectivist rather than an individualistic tradition, and such a perspective places the needs of the family above the needs of the individual; this has important implications for communicating public health messages. There has some been research on cultural communication competency in clinical settings,[49-51] but only limited research in public health situations.[52,53] There is a great need for more qualitative and quantitative research on how to best communicate cross-culturally in public health and to develop evidence-based guidelines for practice.

BUILDING THE INFRASTRUCTURE FOR EQUITABLE ACCESS AND USE OF NEW COMMUNICATION TECHNOLOGIES

Finally, there is a growing need to address the problem of access and use of new communication technologies.[54] There is reason to be concerned about the growing dichotomy between the communication haves and have-nots, or the so-called "digital divide."[23] In the U.S., Internet access and use is common among younger persons and those with higher levels of income and education; although the gap has narrowed, Internet access and use is less common persons who are older, reside in rural areas, have lower levels of education or income, or are African-American or Hispanic.[23,54]

These disadvantaged groups are usually the very populations that public health practitioners most need to reach. It may be tempting to believe that information posted on the World Wide Web effectively reaches everyone, but this is untrue for many audiences. If new communication devices and methods are not accessible to, or understood by, members of vulnerable population groups, they can have little impact on improving health. To address the digital divide effectively, adequate private and public resources are necessary to ensure that new communication technologies are available and can be easily used by everyone.

CONCLUSION

These are exciting but challenging times for public health communication. Given the recent advances in information technologies, there are unprecedented opportunities to communicate information rapidly to multiple audiences. Yet there are great challenges as well, such as overcoming the digital divide, information overload, cross-cultural communication, and understanding the best processes for translating information to nonscientific audiences in the United States and elsewhere to improve health. There is a great and ongoing need to better understand how to take advantage of opportunities to communicate public health information.

CHAPTER 14 ENDNOTES

1. Terris M. The complex tasks of the second epidemiologic revolution: The Joseph W. Mountin Lecture. *J Public Health Policy.* 1983;4:8-24.
2. Susser M, Susser E. Choosing a future for epidemiology: I. Eras and paradigms. *Am J Public Health.* 1996;86:668-673.
3. Leet T, Weidner S, Brownson R. *Assessing the competencies and training needs of state and territorial chronic disease program staff.* Final Report prepared for the Association of State and Territorial Chronic Disease Program Directors. St. Louis, MO: Saint Louis University School of Public Health; 2001.
4. Institute of Medicine. *The Future of Public Health.* Washington, DC: National Academy Press; 1988.
5. Shy CM. The failure of academic epidemiology: witness for the prosecution. *Am J Epidemiol.* 1997;145(6):479-84.
6. Brownson RC, Kreuter MW. Future trends affecting public health: challenges and opportunities. *J Public Health Management Practice.* 1997;3:49-60.
7. Loos GP. Minimum competencies for public health personnel. *Asia Pac J Public Health.* 1995;8:195-200.
8. Kreps GL, Bonaguro EW, Query JL. The history and development of the field of health communication. In: Jackson LD, Duffy BK, eds. *Health Communication Research: A Guide to Developments and Directions.* Westport, CT: Greenwood Press; 1998.
9. Siegel M, Doner L. *Marketing Public Health: Strategies to Promote Social Change.* Gaithersburg, MD: Aspen; 1998.
10. Wallack L, Dorfman L, Jernigan D, Themba M. *Media Advocacy and Public Health.* Newbury Park, CA: Sage; 1993.
11. Council on Linkages Between Academia and Public Health Practice. *Consensus Set of Core Competencies.* Washington, DC: Public Health Foundation, 2001. Available at: http://trainingfinder.org/competencies. Date of access: June 22, 2002.
12. Liang AP, Renard PG, Robinson C, Richards TB. Survey of leadership skills needed for state and territorial health officers, United States, 1988. *Public Health Rep.* 1988;108:116-120.
13. Reder S, Gale GL, Taylor J. Using a dual method needs assessment to evaluate the training needs of public health professionals. *J Public Health Management Practice.* 1999;5:62-69.
14. Bone L, Geilen A, Sheciac M, Johnson M, Farfel M, Burke T, Guyer B, Armenian H, Zeger S. *Community-based public health competencies.* Baltimore, MD: The Johns Hopkins University; 1996.
15. Wright K, Rowitz L, Merkle A, Reid WM, Robinson G, Herzog B, et al. Competency development in public health leadership. *Am J Public Health.* 2000;90:1202-1206.
16. Clark NM, Weist E. Mastering the new public health. *Am J Public Health.* 2000;90:1208-1211.
17. Lloyd P. Management competencies in health for all/new public health settings. *J Health Admin.* 1994;12:187-203.
18. The National Public Health Leadership Network for State and Regional Leadership Programs. Public health leadership competency framework, 1997. Available at: http://www.slu.edu/

organizations/nln/news.html. Date of access: June 22, 2002.

19. Association of State and Territorial Health Officials. *Performance Measurement and Assessment Tools.* Washington, DC: Association of State and Territorial Health Officials, 2002. Available at: http://www.astho.org/phiip/performance.html. Date of access: June 22, 2002.

20. Potter MA, Pistella CL, Fertman CI, Dato VM. Needs assessment and a model agenda for training the public health workforce. *Am J Public Health.* 2000;90:1294-1296.

21. Centers for Disease Control and Prevention. *CDCynergy 2001.* Atlanta, GA: Centers for Disease Control and Prevention, 2001.

22. 8th Annual Tobacco Use Prevention Training Institute, July 2002. Chapel Hill, NC: Tobacco Use Prevention Training Institute Program. Available at: http://www.tupti.org. Date of access: June 22, 2002.

23. Science Panel on Interactive Communication and Health. *Wired for Health and Well-Being: the Emergence of Interactive Health Communication.* Eng TR, Gustafson DH, eds. Washington DC: US Department of Health and Human Services; 1999.

24. U.S. Department of Commerce. *A Nation On-line: How Americans Are Expanding Their Use of the Internet.* Washington, DC: U.S. Department of Commerce, Economics and Statistics Administration, National Telecommunications and Information Administration, 2002.

25. Harris Poll. Explosive growth of "cyberchondriacs" continues. Harris Poll #44. New York: Harris Poll, August 11, 2000.

26. National Cancer Institute. *Evidence-Based Guidelines on Web Design and Usability.* Available at: http://usability.gov/guidelines/index.html. Date of access: June 22, 2002.

27. Eysenbach G, Köhler C. How do consumers search for and appraise health information on the world wide web? Qualitative study using focus groups, usability tests, and in-depth interviews. *Br Med J.* 2002; 324:573-577.

28. Meric F, Bernstam EV, Mirza NQ, Hunt KK, Ames FC, Merrick IR, Kuerer HM, Pollock RE, Musen MA, Singletary SE. Breast cancer on the world wide web: cross sectional survey of quality of information and popularity of websites. *Br Med J.* 2002;324:577-581.

29. Thacker SB, Berkelman RL. Public health surveillance in the United States. *Epidemiol Rev.* 1988;10:164-190.

30. Bloom Y, Figgs LW, Baker EA, et al. Data uses, benefits and barriers of the Behavioral Risk Factor Surveillance System: a qualitative study. *J Public Health Management Practice.* 2000;6:78-86.

31. Figgs LW, Bloom Y, Dugbatey K, Dugbatey K, Stanwyck C, Nelson DE, Brownson RC. Uses of Behavioral Risk Factor Surveillance System Data, 1993-1997 *Am J Public Health.* 2000;90:774-776.

32. National Cancer Institute. Centers of Excellence in Cancer Communications Research. Available at: http://dccps.nci.nih.gov/communicationcenters/. Date of access: June 22, 2002.

33. U.S. Department of Health and Human Services. *Preventing Tobacco Use Among Young People: A Report of the Surgeon General.* Atlanta, GA: U.S. Department of Health and Human Services, Public Health Service, Centers for Disease Control and Prevention, National Center for Chronic Disease Prevention and Health Promotion, Office on Smoking and Health; 1994.

34. U.S. Department of Health and Human Services. 10th *Special Report to the U.S. Congress on Alcohol and Health.* Bethesda, MD: National Institute on Alcohol Abuse and Alcoholism; 2000. Available at: http://www.niaaa.nih.gov/publications/10report/intro.pdf. Date of access: June 22, 2002.

35. American Cancer Society. *Cancer Facts and Figures, 2001.* Available at: http://www3.cancer.org/cancerinfo/. Date of access: June 22, 2002.

36. U.S. Preventive Services Task Force. *Guide to Clinical Preventive Services.* Baltimore, MD: Williams and Wilkins; 1996.

37. Zaza S, Carande-Kulis VG, Sleet DA, Sosin DM, Elder RW, Shults RA, Dinh-Zarr TB, Nichols JL, Thompson RS. Methods for conducting systematic reviews of the evidence of effectiveness and economic efficiency of interventions to reduce injuries to motor vehicle occupants. *Am J Prev Med.* 2001; 21(4 Suppl):23-30.

38. National Institutes of Health Consensus Development Program. Available at: http://odp.od.nih.gov/consensus.

39. Kohn LT, Corrigan JM, Donaldson MS, eds. *To Err is Human.* Washington, DC: Committee on Quality of Health Care in America, Institute of Medicine; 2000.

40. National Cancer Institute Web site: http://www.cancer.gov. Date of access; June 22, 2002.
41. Centers for Disease Control and Prevention Web site: http://www.cdc.gov. Date of access: June 22, 2002.
42. Woolf SH. The need for perspective in evidence-based medicine. *JAMA.* 1999;282:2358-2365.
43. Slater MD. Choosing audience segmentation strategies and methods for health communication. In: Maibach E, Parrott R, eds. *Designing Health Messages: Approaches from Communication Theory and Practice.* Thousand Oaks, CA: Sage; 1995: 186-198.
44. McQuail D. *Mass Communication Theory: An Introduction,* 4th ed. London: Sage; 2000.
45. U.S. Bureau of the Census. *Statistical Abstract of the United States: 2001.* Washington, DC: U.S. Census Bureau; 2001.
46. Gudykunst WB, Mody B. *Handbook of International and Intercultural Communication.* 2nd Ed. Thousand Oaks, CA: Sage; 2002.
47. Tanjasiri S, Wallace SP, Shibata K. Picture imperfect: hidden problems among Asian and Pacific Islander elderly. *Gerontologist.* 1995;35:752-650.
48. Centers for Disease Control and Prevention. *Reported Tuberculosis in the United States, 2000.* Atlanta, GA: National Center for HIV, STD, and TB Prevention, 2001.
49. Cooper-Patrick L, Gallo J, Gonzales JJ, Vu HT, Powe NR, Nelson C, Ford DE. Race, gender, and partnership in the patient-physician relationship. *JAMA.* 1999;282:583-589.
50. McLauglin LA, Braun KL. Asian and Pacific Islander cultural values: considerations for health care decision making. *Health Social Work.* 1998;23:116-127.
51. Helton LR. Intervention with Appalachians: strategies for a culturally specific practice. *J Cultural Diversity.* 1995;2:20-26.
52. Weeks MR, Schensul JJ, Williams SS, Singer M, Grier M. AIDS-prevention for African-American and Latina women—building culturally and gender-appropriate intervention. *AIDS Educ Prev.* 1995;7:251-264.
53. Dushay RA, Singer M, Weeks MR, Rohena L, Gruber R. Lowering HIV risk among ethnic minority drug users: comparing culturally targeted intervention to a standard intervention. *Am J Drug Alcohol Abuse.* 2001;27:501-524.
54. Dickard N. *Federal retrenchment on the digital divide: potential national impact.* Washington, DC: Benton Foundation, Policy Brief #1, March 2002.

SUGGESTED READINGS AND RESOURCES

Brownson RC, Kreuter MW. Future trends affecting public health: challenges and opportunities. *J Public Health Management Practice.* 1997;3:49-60.

Centers for Disease Control and Prevention. *CDCynergy 2001.* Atlanta, GA: Centers for Disease Control and Prevention; 2001.

Reder S, Gale GL, Taylor J. Using a dual method needs assessment to evaluate the training needs of public health professionals. *J Public Health Management Practice.* 1999;5:62-69.

Siegel M, Doner L. *Marketing Public Health: Strategies to Promote Social Change.* Gaithersburg, MD: Aspen; 1998.

Woolf SH. The need for perspective in evidence-based medicine. *JAMA.* 1999;282:2358-2365.

STEP-BY STEP PLANNING GUIDE FOR COMMUNICATING PUBLIC HEALTH INFORMATION

1. WHAT IS THE SCIENTIFIC EVIDENCE?

Describe the problem to be addressed, the strength of the scientific evidence, and the extent of scientific consensus behind the communication activity:

_____

_____

_____

2. WHY IS COMMUNICATION NECESSARY (PURPOSE)?

- Inform individuals
- Inform policy makers (administrator or elected officials)
- Persuade individuals (e.g., to change attitudes or behaviors)
- Persuade policy makers

The specific purpose of this activity is to:

_____

_____

_____

3. WHO IS THE AUDIENCE?

A. PRIMARY AUDIENCE

- General Public (specify):_____
- Administrator (specify):_____
- Elected official(s) (specify):_____
- Voluntary health organization(s) (specify):_____

- Private health organization(s) (specify):_____
- Health care providers (specify):_____
- News media (specify):_____
- Other (specify):_____

B. SECONDARY OR TERTIARY AUDIENCE

- General Public (specify):_____
- Administrator (specify):_____
- Elected official(s) (specify):_____
- Voluntary health organization (s) (specify):_____
- Private health organization (s) (specify):_____
- Health care providers (specify):_____
- News media (specify):_____
- Other (specify):_____

4. WHAT IS THE MESSAGE?

The message concept is the main idea to convey to the audience should be condensed to one or two sentences.   Exact wording for the final message needs to be developed and pretested with content experts and members of the intended audience.

Pretesting of message with technical experts (specify who and when):

_____

Pretesting of message wording and delivery formats with persons from intended audience(s) (specify who and when):

_____

Main Message:

_____
_____
_____

Supporting Messages:

_____
_____
_____

5. HOW AND WHERE SHOULD THE MESSAGE BE DELIVERED?
(SELECT ALL THAT WILL BE USED)

- Written communication (specify):_____
- Visual communication (specify):_____
- Oral presentation
- Electronic communication (specify):_____
- Interpersonal communication (e.g., phone call, face-to-face meeting)
- Mass media (specify): _____

6. WHEN SHOULD THE MESSAGE BE DELIVERED?

Reactive communication. Consider the deadline specified by the requestor, the individual or organization requesting information, effort and resources needed to reply, and competing priorities.

Response will occur on or before (date and time):

_____

Proactive communication. Consider the issue, the audience, the amount of existing attention, and competition with other issues.

Communication activities will occur on or about (specify dates for each audience):

_____

_____

7. IMPLEMENT THE COMMUNICATION PLAN

Communication activities that actually occurred and dates:

_____

_____

_____

_____

8. DID THE AUDIENCE RECEIVE THE INFORMATION AND WAS IT EFFECTIVE?

Process evaluation (specify what will be used to measure receipt of communication message by audience): _____

Outcome evaluation (specify what will be used to measure(s) the effectiveness of the communication): _____

OTHER CONSIDERATIONS (E.G., RESOURCES, OTHER PRIORITIES, BARRIERS):

Specify: _____

_____

_____

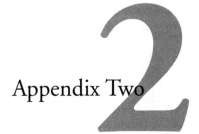

COMMUNICATING PUBLIC HEALTH INFORMATION EFFECTIVELY DIRECTORIES AND OTHER SELECTED INTERNET WEB SITES FOR LOCATING PUBLIC HEALTH DATA

Note: Web site addresses are subject to change without notice

DIRECTORIES

AMERICAN FACTFINDER
http://factfinder.census.gov/servlet/BasicFactsServlet

DIRECTORY OF HEALTH AND HUMAN SERVICES DATA RESOURCES
http://aspe.os.dhhs.gov/datacncl/datadir

FEDERAL INTERAGENCY FORUM ON CHILD AND FAMILY STATISTICS
http://www.childstats.gov

FEDERAL STATISTICS
http://www.fedstats.gov

HEALTHFINDER
http://www.healthfinder.gov

NATIONAL HEALTH INFORMATION CENTER
http://www.health.gov/nhic

SOCIAL STATISTICS BRIEFING ROOM
http://www.whitehouse.gov/fsbr/ssbr.html

WORLD HEALTH ORGANIZATION STATISTICAL INFORMATION SYSTEM (WHOSIS)
http://www.who.int/whosis

HEALTH POLL SEARCH
http://www.kaisernetwork.org/health_poll/hpoll_index.cfm

FEDERAL HEALTH AGENCIES

ADMINSTRATION FOR CHILDREN AND FAMILIES (ACF)
http://www.acf.dhhs.gov

ADMINISTRATION ON AGING (AoA)
http://www.aoa.dhhs.gov

AGENCY FOR HEALTHCARE RESEARCH QUALITY (AHRQ)
http://www.ahrq.gov

AGENCY FOR TOXIC SUBSTANCES AND DISEASE REGISTRY (ATSDR)
http://atsdr1.atsdr.cdc.gov

CENTERS FOR DISEASE CONTROL AND PREVENTION (CDC)
http://www.cdc.gov

CENTER FOR MEDICARE & MEDICAID SERVICES (CMS)
http://www.cms.hhs.gov

DEPARTMENT OF HEALTH AND HUMAN SERVICES (DHHS)
http://dhhs.gov

HEALTH RESOURCES AND SERVICES ADMINISTRATION (HRSA)
http://www.hrsa.gov

INDIAN HEALTH SERVICE (IHS)
http://www.ihs.gov

NATIONAL INSTITUTES OF HEALTH (NIH)
http://www.nih.gov

OFFICE OF DISEASE PREVENTION AND HEALTH PROMOTION
http://www.odphp.osophs.dhhs.gov

OFFICE OF POPULATION AFFAIRS (OPA)
http://opa.osophs.dhhs.gov

OFFICE OF THE ASSISTANT SECRETARY FOR PLANNING AND EVALUATION (OASPE)
http://www.aspe.dhhs.gov

SUBSTANCE ABUSE AND MENTAL HEALTH SERVICES ADMINISTRATION (SAMHSA)
http://www.samhsa.gov

OTHER FEDERAL AGENCIES

AGENCY FOR INTERNATIONAL DEVELOPMENT
http://www.usaid.gov

BUREAU OF THE CENSUS
http://www.census.gov

BUREAU OF JUSTICE STATISTICS
http://www.ojp.usdoj.gov/bjs

BUREAU OF LABOR STATISTICS
http://www.bls.gov

BUREAU OF TRANSPORTATION STATISTICS
http://www.bts.gov

CONSUMER PRODUCT SAFETY COMMISSION
http://cpsc.gov

DEPARTMENT OF VETERANS AFFAIRS (VA)
http://www.va.gov

DRUG ENFORCEMENT ADMINISTRATION
http://www.usdoj.gov/dea

ENVIRONMENTAL PROTECTION AGENCY
http://www.epa.gov

FEDERAL EMERGENCY MANAGEMENT AGENCY
http://www.fema.gov

NATIONAL CENTER FOR EDUCATION STATISTICS
http://nces.ed.gov

NATIONAL HIGHWAY TRAFFIC SAFETY ADMINISTRATION
http://www.nhtsa.dot.gov

OCCUPATIONAL SAFETY AND HEALTH ADMINISTRATION (OSHA)
http://www.osha.gov

OFFICE OF POPULATION AFFAIRS (OPA)
http://opa.osophs.dhhs.gov

UNITED STATES DEPARTMENT OF AGRICULTURE
http://www.usda.gov

OTHER SOURCES

AMERICAN CANCER SOCIETY
http://cancer.org

AMERICAN DIABETES ASSOCIATION
http://www.diabetes.org

AMERICAN HEART ASSOCIATION
http://www.americanheart.org

AMERICAN LUNG ASSOCIATION
http://www.lungusa.org

GUIDE TO COMMUNITY PREVENTIVE SERVICES
http://www.thecommunityguide.org

MONITORING THE FUTURE (HIGH SCHOOL SENIORS) DATA
http://monitoringthefuture.org

NATIONAL GUIDELINE CLEARINGHOUSE
http://www.guideline.gov

UNICEF
http://www.unicef.org

WORLD HEALTH ORGANIZATION (WHO)
http://www.who.int

Appendix Three

INTERNET WEB SITES ADDRESSES FOR HEALTH DEPARTMENTS FOR STATES AND THE DISTRICT OF COLUMBIA STATE OR TERRITORY

Note: Web site addresses are subject to change without notice

ALABAMA
http://www.adph.org

ALASKA
http://health.hss.state.ak.us

ARIZONA
http://www.hs.state.az.us

ARKANSAS
http://www.healthyarkansas.com

CALIFORNIA
http://www.dhs.cahwnet.gov

COLORADO
http://www.cdphe.state.co.us

CONNECTICUT
http://www.dph.state.ct.us

DELAWARE
http://www.state.de.us/dhss/dhss.htm

DISTRICT OF COLUMBIA
http://www.dchealth.gov

FLORIDA
http://www.doh.state.fl.us

GEORGIA
http://www.ph.dhr.state.ga.us

HAWAII
http://www.state.hi.us/health

IDAHO
http://www2.state.id.us/dhw

ILLINOIS
http://www.idph.state.il.us

INDIANA
http://www.state.in.us/isdh

IOWA
http://www.idph.state.ia.us

KANSAS
http://www.kdhe.state.ks.us

KENTUCKY
http://publichealth.state.ky.us

LOUISIANA
http://www.dhh.state.la.us

MAINE
http://www.state.me.us/dhs

MARYLAND
http://www.dhmh.state.md.us.

MASSACHUSETTS
http://www.state.ma.us/dph

MICHIGAN
http://www.michigan.gov/mdch

MINNESOTA
http://www.health.state.mn.us

MISSISSIPPI
http://www.msdh.state.ms.us

MISSOURI
http://www.health.state.mo.us

MONTANA
http://www.dphhs.state.mt.us

NEBRASKA
http://www.hhs.state.ne.us

NEVADA
http://health2k.state.nv.us

NEW HAMPSHIRE
http://www.dhhs.state.nh.us

NEW JERSEY
http://www.state.nj.us/health

NEW MEXICO
http://www.health.state.nm.us

NEW YORK
http://www.health.state.ny.us

NORTH CAROLINA
http://www.dhhs.state.nc.us

NORTH DAKOTA
http://www.health.state.nd.us

OHIO
http://www.odh.state.oh.us

Oklahoma
http://www.health.state.ok.us

OREGON
http://www.ohd.hr.state.or.us

PENNSYLVANIA
http://webserver.health.state.pa.us/health/site

RHODE ISLAND
http://www.health.state.ri.us

SOUTH CAROLINA
http://www.scdhec.net

SOUTH DAKOTA
http://www.state.sd.us/doh

TENNESSEE
http://www.state.tn.us/health

TEXAS
http://www.tdh.state.tx.us

UTAH
http://hlunix.hl.state.ut.us

VERMONT
http://www.state.vt.us/health

VIRGINIA
http://www.vdh.state.va.us

WASHINGTON
http://www.doh.wa.gov

WEST VIRGINIA
http://www.wvdhhr.org

WISCONSIN
http://www.dhfs.state.wi.us

WYOMING
http://wdhfs.state.wy.us/WDH

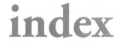
index

Page numbers followed by an "f" or a "t" indicate figures and tables, respectively.

Administrators in public health organizations, 98–99
Advocacy, 61, 84–86
Asbestos risks communication example, 23–24
Audiences
characteristics identification, 15–17
electronic communication considerations, 177
hierarchy of message impact on recipient, 12
information communication and
challenges and barriers, 54–55
channels, 51
culture and language issues, 16, 50–51
informing vs. persuading, 14–15
lack of interest by nonscientists, 4–5
literacy and numeracy (See Literacy and numeracy)
primary, secondary, tertiary, 49–50
segmentation, 15–17, 49
infrastructure access and, 209
oral presentations and, 143
persuasive communication and, 67
policy makers as, 15–16, 101
private and voluntary health organizations as, 118–119, 120
for public health information, 3–4
rank order of relationships, 17
reach of the message and, 21
readiness stage, 17
risk communication considerations, 189
risk perceptions, technical vs. lay, 187–188
tailoring messages to, 208–209
translating public health data for, 39–40
visual communication considerations, 156
written communication considerations, 130, 136, 137t, 138t

Bar charts use in communicating, 43, 157–158, 159–160f
Bioterrorism and communication, 196–197, 200
Bridging in an interview, 84

CDCynergy, 206
Channels of communication
considerations in communicating to inform, 51
described, 19–20
infrastructure and, 209
media (See News media)
persuasive communication and, 68
recommendations for, 208–209
Color and shading and visual communication, 166–167
Correspondence with elected officials, 110, 111t
Council on Linkages Between Academia and Public Health Practice (2001), 7, 206
Credibility of public health practitioners
News media and, 79
private and voluntary health organizations and, 118
quality of the science assessment and, 37
Culture and language
audience considerations, 16
information communication considerations, 50–51
need for communication improvement, 209

Databases
improvement need, 207–208
locating useful sites, 213–216
for searching public health literature, 34
for target audience information, 17
Data-ink ratio and visual communication, 165–166
Data translation. See Translating public health data
Demographics. See Audiences

Diffusion of Innovations, 65–66
Disease information dissemination, 121–122

Educational approaches to communication, 59–61
Education and training in communication, 205–206
Education reports, 129
Elaboration Likelihood Model (ELM), 52
Elected officials
  characteristics of, 99–100
  recommendations for communicating with
    correspondence, 110, 111t
    face-to-face meetings, 109–110
    factors and approaches overview, 107, 108t, 109
    information presentation considerations, 109
    oral presentations, 109–110
Electronic communication
  background and benefits to use, 173–174
  e-mail recommendations, 178
  information dissemination/gathering, 176
  interventions to persuade, 68, 177
  limitations, 181–182
  networking, 176
  purpose, audience, and message, 177–178
  summary, 182
  surveys for data collection, 175–176
  telemedicine, 177
  types of uses, 175t
  Web sites recommendations
    design and usability, 180–181
    locating useful sites, 178–179, 213–216
    quality of information considerations, 179
ELM (Elaboration Likelihood Model), 52
E-mail and communication, 178
Ethical problems in data presentation, 38
Ethos and oral communication, 143–144

Face-to-face meetings with elected officials, 109–110
Federal Acquisition Streamlining Amendment (FASA, 1998), 119
Fill patterns and visual communication, 167
Framing, message, 67–68

Health communication field, 6–8, 205–206
Health departments Web sites, 217–220

Hierarchy of Effects Model, 21

Individuals as the intended audience, 15–16
Information communication
  audiences and
    challenges and barriers, 54–55
    channels, 51
    culture and language issues, 50–51
    literacy and numeracy (See Literacy and numeracy)
    primary, secondary, tertiary, 49–50
    segmentation, 15–17, 49
  by electronic means (See Electronic communication)
  information processing implications, 52–53
  infrastructure and, 209
  message development and planning, 53–54
  nature of process, 48
  oral presentations and, 142
  for private/voluntary organizations
    audience reach, 118–119
    desire to achieve an objective, 117–118
    influence on organizational development, 119–120
    influence on political process, 119
    requirements, 48–49
    summary, 55
Information technology. See Electronic communication
Internet. See Electronic communication; Web sites

Labels and visual communication, 167–168
Language issues in communication. See Culture and language
Legends and visual communication, 168
Line graphs and visual communication, 158, 161f
Literacy and numeracy
  data presentation example, 103, 104f, 105f
  News media and, 84
  of nonscientific audiences, 5, 40–41, 50
  numeric analogies use, 41, 42t
  writing for low literacy, 136, 137t, 138t

Maps
  for media presentations, 86, 88–93f
  for translating public health data, 43
  for visual communication, 160, 162f

Marketing and communicating to persuade, 61

Mass media. See News media

Mathematical literacy. See Literacy and numeracy

Measles outbreak communication example, 24–26

Media. See News media

Media advocacy, 84–86

Message
development and testing, 17–18, 19t
electronic communication considerations, 177–178
framing, 67–68
hierarchy impact on recipient, 12
for informative communication, 53–54
media and channels, 18–20
oral presentations considerations, 144–146
in persuasive communication, 66–67, 68–69
policy makers, considerations for, 101
private and voluntary health organizations and, 121
production and delivery to policy makers, 76, 102
reach and the audience, 21
risk communication considerations, 189–190
tailoring to audiences, 208–209
timing considerations, 20
visual communication considerations, 156
written communication considerations, 130

News media
agenda setting, 74–75
attention getting example, 86, 88–93
challenges and barriers, 86–87
characteristics and recommendations
appropriateness of communication, 80
business aspects and competition, 76–77
differences among media forms, 80
help from experienced people, 80–81
newsworthiness determination, 78–79
relationships with reporters, 79
science vs. news, 77–78
forms and reach of media, 74
interview recommendations
literacy and numeracy considerations, 84
preparation, 81
SOHCO development and use, 76, 82–83
sufficiency of answers, 84

tips for, 85t
media advocacy, 84–86
message considerations, 76
practitioners' inexperience with, 5
reactive or proactive purpose, 75–76
summary, 94
timing considerations, 76

Numeracy, 50. See also Literacy and numeracy

Obesity study media presentation example, 86, 88–93f

Oral presentations
audience considerations, 143
challenges and barriers, 152–153
delivery, 147–148
for elected officials, 109–110
feedback, 149–150
language, 146–147
message considerations, 144–146
persuasive speech outline example, 145t
purpose considerations, 142, 145t, 146
recommendations for improving, 150–152
speaker's image, 143–144
summary, 153
types of oral communication, 141–142
visual aids use, 149

Persuasive communication
approaches and theories
Diffusion of Innovations, 65–66
Precede-Proceed Model, 62–63
Social Cognitive Theory, 63
Stages-of-Change, 64–65
Theory of Planned Behavior, 64
Theory of Reasoned Action, 63–64
audience considerations, 67
channels, 68
cost/benefit approach, 59–61
by electronic means, 68, 177
message evaluation, 68–69
message framing, 67–68
oral presentations and, 142, 145t, 146
purpose considerations, 66
social marketing, 60–61
summary, 69

Philip Morris, 117–118

Pictures and visual communication, 160, 162, 163f

Pie charts

for translating public health data, 43
visual communication and, 158, 161f
Planning public health communication
case examples
asbestos risks, 23–24
measles outbreak, 24–26
resource advocation, 27–28
SIDS prevention, 22–23
tobacco access by youths, 26–27
hierarchy of message impact on recipient, 12
for risk communication, 196, 197t, 198–200f
steps involved
assessing the science/translating data, 13–14
audience characteristics identification, 15–17
evaluation, 21
implementation, 20–21
message development and testing, 17–18, 19t
message media and channels, 18–20
message timing, 18–20
overview, 12–13
purpose definition, 14–15
summary, 28–29
Policy assessments, 130
Policy makers
audience considerations, 101
background to policy makers' role, 97–98
challenges and barriers, 111–112
characteristics of administrators, 98–99
characteristics of elected officials, 99–100
as the intended audience, 15–16, 101
message considerations, 101–102
public health vs. political decision-making, 98, 99t
purpose considerations, 100
recommendations for, elected officials
correspondence, 110, 111t
face-to-face meetings, 109–110
factors and approaches overview, 107, 108t, 109
information presentation, 109
oral presentations, 109–110
recommendations for, general, 102–105, 106f
spokesperson selection, 102
summary, 112
Position papers, 130
Precede-Proceed Model, 62–63
Pre-testing of messages, 53–54

Primary audiences, 17, 49–50
Private and voluntary health organizations
audience considerations, 120
challenges and barriers, 123–124
exchange negotiation, 122–123
influence on public health, 115–116
message considerations, 121
private health organizations description, 116–117
purpose considerations, 120
rationale for communicating information to
audience reach, 118–119
desire to achieve an objective, 117–118
influence on organizational development, 119–120
influence on political process, 119
summary, 125
types of data to communicate, 121–122
voluntary health organizations description, 117
Public health communication planning. See
Planning public health communication
Public health information
audiences for, 3–4
barriers to communication, 4–5
cultural considerations, 209
definitions, 3
education and training for communicating, 205–206
importance of communicating, 1–2
infrastructure access considerations, 209–210
message and channel considerations, 208–209
research need, 206–207
translation need, 207–208

Resource advocation communication example, 27–28
Risk communication
bioterrorism and, 196–197, 200
categories, 186–187
challenges and barriers, 194–196
education goal, 188–189
motivation for and approaches to, 185–186
perceptions of risk, technical vs. lay audience, 187–188
planning for, 196, 197t, 198–200f
purpose, audience, and message, 189–190
recommendations for
audience fear and anger issues, 191
multiple perspectives considerations, 191–192

necessity consideration, 191
resources and personnel, 192
risk assessments, 191
situational uniqueness realization, 190
specificity about action, 194
stakeholders involvement, 192
translating the science, 193–194
uncertainty acknowledgement, 193
terms used, 186
types of tasks, 186

Secondary audiences, 17, 49–50
Segmentation, audience, 15–17, 49
Self-efficacy, 63
SIDS prevention
communication example, 22–23
information communication example, 60
Single overriding health communication
objective (SOHCO)
message content and development, 17–18
News media and, 76, 82–83
Social Cognitive Theory, 63
Social marketing and persuasive communica-
tion, 60–61
SOHCO. See Single overriding health com-
munication objective
Special reports, 129–130
Stages-of-Change, 64–65
Surveys for data collection, 175–176

Tables and visual communication, 157
Technical reports/publications, 128
Telemedicine, 177
Tertiary audiences, 17, 49–50
Theory of Planned Behavior, 64
Theory of Reasoned Action, 63–64
Titles and visual communication, 167
Tobacco access by youths communication
example, 26–27
Tobacco Use Prevention Training Institute
(TUPTI), 206
Translating public health data
audience interest considerations, 39–40
challenges and barriers, 43
ethical presentation of data, 38
improvement need, 207–208
literacy and numeracy considerations, 40–41
locating information, 33–36
numeric analogies use, 41, 42t

quality assessment, 37–38
recommended formats, 42–43
for risk communication, 193–194
selective use of data, 38–39
summary, 43–44
in written communication, 135t
Typography considerations and visual communication, 164–165

Visual aids use in oral presentations, 149
Visual communication
bar charts, 157–158, 159–160f
challenges and barriers, 168–169, 170f
color and shading, 166–167
considerations, 156
data-ink ratio, 165–166
elements, 155
fill patterns, 167
labels, 167–168
legends, 168
line graphs, 158, 161f
maps, 160, 162f
pictures, 160, 162, 163f
pie charts, 158, 161f
purpose, audience, and message, 156
summary, 169, 171
tables, 157
titles, 167
types summary, 157t
typography considerations, 164–165
Voluntary health organizations. See Private and
voluntary health organizations

Web sites. See also Electronic communication
bioterrorism, 200
design and usability, 180–181
health departments, 217–220
locating useful sites, 178–179, 213–216
quality of information considerations, 179
for searching public health literature, 34t,
35–36t
Written communication
content recommendations, 132–134
general recommendations, 131–132
for low literacy audiences, 136, 137t, 138t
purpose, audience, and message, 130
style recommendations, 134
summary, 136, 138
translating public health terms, 135t

types used, 128t
  educational reports, 129
  special reports, 129–130
  technical reports/publications, 128